GOUT DIET COOKBOOK

Gout Diet Guidebook: Easy Low-Purine Recipes, Family-friendly Recipes, Meal Preparation Strategies and Meal Plans for Managing Gout and Reducing Uric Acid.

Isabella C. James

GOUT DIET COOKBOOK

All rights reserved. No part of this publication may be reproduced, distributed, or transmitted in any form or by any means, including photocopying, recording, or other electronic or mechanical methods, without the prior written permission of the publisher, except in the case of brief quotations embodied in critical reviews and certain other noncommercial uses permitted by copyright law.

Copyright © Isabella C. James, 2024.

TABLE OF CONTENT

CHAPTER ONE

INTRODUCTION

1.1 Understanding Gout

Gout. It's a word that might bring to mind images of medieval kings, overindulgence, and painful joints. But what exactly is gout, and why should we be concerned about it today? Let's delve into the basics of this ancient ailment that still affects millions of people around the world.

Gout is a type of arthritis, a condition that causes pain and inflammation in the joints. Unlike other forms of arthritis, gout has a unique and very specific cause: the buildup of uric acid in the body. Uric acid is a waste product that comes from the breakdown of substances called purines, which are found in many of the foods we eat and also produced naturally by the body. Under normal circumstances, uric acid dissolves in the blood and passes through the kidneys into the urine. However, when the body produces too much uric acid or doesn't eliminate enough of it, the acid can form sharp, needle-like crystals in the joints. These crystals trigger the severe pain and inflammation characteristic of a gout attack.

Imagine you're enjoying a perfectly fine day, and suddenly, out of nowhere, a joint—often the big toe—becomes excruciatingly painful, swollen, and red. This is what a gout flare feels like, and it can be debilitating. While the big toe is the classic site of a gout attack, other joints such as the ankles, knees, wrists, and fingers can also be affected. The pain can be so intense that even the light touch of a bedsheet can feel unbearable.

But gout isn't just about pain. Over time, repeated gout attacks can lead to chronic arthritis, joint damage, and even kidney stones. This is why it's essential to manage gout effectively, not just to relieve the immediate pain but to prevent long-term complications.

The Role of Diet in Gout

So, where does diet come into play? Since gout is directly related to the levels of uric acid in the body, and uric acid comes from the breakdown of purines, the foods we eat have a significant impact on gout. Certain foods are high in purines and can increase uric acid levels, triggering gout attacks. These include red meat, organ meats, and certain types of seafood. Alcohol, especially beer, is another big culprit. On the other hand, some foods can help reduce uric acid levels or prevent gout attacks.

Adopting a gout-friendly diet can make a world of difference. It's not just about avoiding certain foods but also about embracing a healthy, balanced diet that supports overall well-being. For instance, low-fat dairy products, whole grains, and plenty of fruits and vegetables are excellent choices. Hydration is also key—drinking plenty of water helps flush uric acid from the body.

Beyond Diet: A Holistic Approach

While diet is crucial, managing gout often requires a holistic approach. Maintaining a healthy weight, staying physically active, and taking medications prescribed by a healthcare provider can all play vital roles in controlling gout. Stress management and good sleep hygiene are also important, as stress and lack of sleep can trigger flare-ups.

A Personal Journey

Every person with gout has their own story. For some, the journey with gout starts with a single, inexplicable attack. For others, it's a gradual realization as joint pain becomes more frequent and severe. Whatever the case, understanding gout is the first step towards managing it effectively. This book aims to be your companion on this journey, offering not just recipes but also practical tips and insights to help you live a full, active life despite gout.

As you read through this cookbook, remember that managing gout is a marathon, not a sprint. It requires patience, persistence, and a willingness to make changes. But with the right tools and knowledge, you can take control of your health and minimize the impact of gout on your life. Let's embark on this journey together, starting with understanding what gout is and how we can manage it through the power of food.

1.2 The Role of Diet in Managing Gout

Diet plays a pivotal role in managing gout, a condition deeply intertwined with what we eat and drink. The foods and beverages we consume can significantly influence the levels of uric acid in our blood, which, in turn, can trigger or prevent gout attacks. Let's explore how dietary choices impact gout and how a well-planned diet can help manage this condition effectively.

Understanding Purines and Uric Acid

To understand how diet affects gout, we first need to delve into purines and uric acid. Purines are natural substances found in many foods and are also produced by the body. When purines are broken down, they produce uric acid, which is usually dissolved in the blood, filtered by the kidneys, and excreted in the urine. However, when the body produces too much uric acid or doesn't eliminate enough of it, uric acid levels build up, leading to the formation of sharp, needle-like crystals in the joints. This is what causes the intense pain and inflammation of a gout attack.

Foods to Avoid

Certain foods are high in purines and can increase the risk of gout attacks. Here are some foods to steer clear of:

- ✓ **Red Meat:** Beef, lamb, and pork are all high in purines and can raise uric acid levels.

- ✓ **Organ Meats:** Liver, kidneys, and other organ meats contain extremely high levels of purines.

- ✓ **Certain Seafood:** Shellfish (like shrimp, crab, and lobster) and oily fish (like anchovies, sardines, and mackerel) are rich in purines.

- ✓ **Alcohol:** Beer, in particular, is high in purines and can increase uric acid production. Other alcoholic beverages can also contribute to dehydration, which can exacerbate gout symptoms.

✓ **Sugary Foods and Beverages:** Foods and drinks high in sugar, especially those sweetened with high-fructose corn syrup, can increase uric acid levels.

Foods to Limit

While some foods should be avoided altogether, others should be consumed in moderation:

✓ **Certain Vegetables:** Asparagus, spinach, cauliflower, and mushrooms are moderately high in purines. However, the benefits of these vegetables often outweigh the risks, so they can be included in the diet in reasonable amounts.

✓ **Yeast and Yeast Extracts:** Found in supplements and certain foods, these can also be moderately high in purines.

Foods to Include

Incorporating the right foods into your diet can help manage gout by lowering uric acid levels and reducing inflammation. Here are some beneficial choices:

✓ **Low-fat Dairy Products:** Milk, yogurt, and cheese can help lower uric acid levels and are good sources of protein.

- ✓ **Fruits and Vegetables:** A diet rich in fruits and vegetables provides essential vitamins and antioxidants. Cherries, in particular, have been shown to reduce the frequency of gout attacks.

- ✓ **Whole Grains:** Brown rice, whole wheat bread, and oatmeal are excellent sources of fiber and can help with overall health.

- ✓ **Water:** Staying well-hydrated helps flush uric acid from the body, reducing the risk of crystal formation in the joints.

- ✓ **Lean Proteins:** Chicken, turkey, and tofu are good alternatives to red meat and organ meats.

Hydration and Gout

Hydration plays a critical role in managing gout. Drinking plenty of water helps dilute uric acid and supports the kidneys in excreting it from the body. Aim for at least 8-12 cups of water a day, and more if you're physically active or live in a hot climate.

Beyond Diet: A Comprehensive Approach

While diet is a cornerstone of gout management, it's not the only factor. Maintaining a healthy weight is crucial, as excess weight can increase uric acid production. Regular physical activity helps keep the joints flexible and supports overall health. Additionally, medications prescribed by a healthcare provider can help control uric acid levels and manage pain during gout attacks.

Personalizing Your Gout Diet

Every individual is unique, and what works for one person might not work for another. It's essential to tailor your diet to your specific needs and preferences. Keeping a food diary can help you track which foods trigger your gout symptoms and which ones don't. Working with a dietitian can also provide personalized guidance and support.

Dietary changes can make a significant difference in managing gout. By avoiding high-purine foods, embracing low-purine alternatives, and staying well-hydrated, you can reduce your risk of painful gout attacks and improve your overall quality of life. Remember, managing gout is a journey, and every step you take towards healthier eating is a step towards a more comfortable and active life.

1.3 Purpose of This Cookbook

Living with gout can be a challenging experience, with its sudden and excruciating flare-ups disrupting daily life. Managing gout effectively requires a multifaceted approach, and diet plays a crucial role in this. The purpose of this cookbook is to provide you with the knowledge, tools, and delicious recipes you need to take control of your health and reduce the impact of gout on your life.

Empowering You with Knowledge

Understanding the connection between diet and gout is the first step towards effective management. This cookbook aims to demystify the science behind gout, explaining how certain foods and beverages can trigger or prevent gout attacks. By providing clear, accessible information, we hope to empower you to make informed dietary choices that will help manage your condition.

Providing Practical Solutions

Managing a health condition through diet can often feel overwhelming, especially with the abundance of conflicting information out there. This cookbook is designed to cut through the noise and offer practical, evidence-based solutions. From detailed lists of foods to avoid and include to comprehensive meal plans, we've got you covered. Our goal is to make it as easy as possible for you to adopt a gout-friendly diet without feeling deprived or restricted.

Delicious and Nutritious Recipes

One of the biggest misconceptions about a therapeutic diet is that it has to be bland and boring. This cookbook aims to shatter that myth by offering a wide variety of delicious and nutritious recipes that are both gout-friendly and satisfying. Whether you're looking for hearty breakfasts, light lunches, comforting dinners, or tasty snacks, you'll find plenty of options to suit your tastes and needs. Each recipe is crafted to be flavorful, enjoyable, and easy to prepare, proving that a gout-friendly diet can be both nutritious and delicious.

Supporting Long-term Health

Gout management isn't just about avoiding flare-ups; it's about supporting your long-term health and well-being. This cookbook emphasizes a balanced, holistic approach to diet that promotes overall health. By incorporating a variety of nutrient-dense foods and staying hydrated, you'll not only manage gout more effectively but also support your overall health, energy levels, and vitality.

GOUT DIET COOKBOOK

Flexibility and Personalization

We understand that everyone's journey with gout is unique, and dietary needs and preferences can vary widely. This cookbook is designed with flexibility in mind, offering options for different dietary restrictions and preferences, including vegetarian, vegan, gluten-free, and dairy-free recipes. We encourage you to experiment with the recipes, adapt them to your tastes, and find what works best for your body.

Building a Community

Managing a chronic condition can sometimes feel isolating, but you're not alone. This cookbook is part of a larger effort to build a supportive community of individuals who understand what it's like to live with gout. By sharing your experiences, tips, and favorite recipes, you can connect with others on the same journey and find encouragement and inspiration along the way.

The purpose of this cookbook is to be a valuable resource on your journey towards better health and gout management. By offering comprehensive information, practical solutions, and delicious recipes, we aim to help you take control of your diet and reduce the impact of gout on your life. Remember, managing gout is a marathon, not a sprint, and every small step you take towards healthier eating is a step towards a more comfortable and fulfilling life. Let this cookbook be your guide and companion as you navigate the path to better health.

CHAPTER TWO

GETTING STARTED

2.1 Essential Kitchen Tools for a Gout-Friendly Diet

Embarking on the journey to manage gout through diet is an empowering step. One of the first things you'll need to do is equip your kitchen with the right tools. Having the proper kitchen gadgets can make meal preparation more efficient, enjoyable, and effective in supporting your health goals. Let's dive into the essential kitchen tools that will help you create delicious, gout-friendly meals.

1. Sharp Knives

A good set of sharp knives is the cornerstone of any kitchen. Whether you're chopping vegetables, slicing fruits, or preparing lean meats, a sharp knife ensures precision and safety. Dull knives can slip and cause accidents, while sharp knives make cutting tasks faster and more efficient. Invest in a high-quality chef's knife, a paring knife, and a serrated knife for all your cutting needs.

2. Cutting Boards

Cutting boards are indispensable for safe and hygienic food preparation. It's a good idea to have separate cutting boards for different types of food to avoid cross-contamination. Use one board for meats and another for fruits and vegetables. Opt for boards that are easy to clean and maintain, such as bamboo or plastic.

3. Measuring Cups and Spoons

Accurate measurements are crucial, especially when following recipes that require precise ingredient ratios. Measuring cups and spoons ensure you're using the right amounts of ingredients, which is important for both the success of your recipes and managing portion sizes. Look for sets that include both dry and liquid measures.

4. Blender and Food Processor

Blenders and food processors are versatile tools that can make meal preparation easier and more enjoyable. A high-quality blender is perfect for making smoothies, which are an excellent way to incorporate more fruits and vegetables into your diet. A food processor can handle tasks like chopping, slicing, and pureeing, saving you time and effort in the kitchen.

5. Steamer Basket

Steaming is one of the healthiest ways to cook vegetables, preserving their nutrients and flavor without adding extra fats or oils. A steamer basket is an inexpensive tool that fits into most pots, allowing you to steam vegetables, fish, and other foods quickly and efficiently.

6. Non-Stick Cookware

Non-stick pots and pans are a great investment for preparing gout-friendly meals. They allow you to cook with less oil, reducing the fat content of your dishes. Look for high-quality non-stick cookware that is durable and easy to clean. A good non-stick skillet and saucepan are essential for everyday cooking.

7. Slow Cooker

A slow cooker can be a lifesaver for busy days when you don't have time to stand over the stove. It allows you to prepare healthy, gout-friendly meals with minimal effort. Simply add your ingredients in the morning, and by dinner time, you'll have a delicious, ready-to-eat meal. Slow cookers are perfect for soups, stews, and lean meat dishes.

8. Spiralizer

A spiralizer is a fun and useful tool that turns vegetables like zucchini, carrots, and sweet potatoes into noodle-like strands. This is a great way to create low-purine, vegetable-based alternatives to pasta, which can be both delicious and satisfying. Spiralized veggies are perfect for salads, stir-fries, and as a base for sauces.

9. Storage Containers

Having a variety of storage containers is essential for meal planning and leftovers. Choose containers that are BPA-free, microwave-safe, and easy to clean. Clear containers allow you to see what's inside at a glance, making it easier to keep track of your meals and snacks. Glass containers are a great option for reheating food without the risk of plastic leaching.

10. Kitchen Scale

A kitchen scale is a handy tool for measuring portions accurately, which is important for managing gout. It can help you control the amount of protein you consume, ensuring you stay within recommended limits. Scales are also useful for baking and following recipes that require precise measurements.

Tips for Setting Up Your Kitchen

- ✓ **Organize Your Space:** Keep your kitchen tidy and organized to make meal preparation more efficient. Store frequently used items within easy reach and keep your countertops clutter-free.

✓ **Stock Up on Essentials:** Keep a supply of gout-friendly pantry staples like whole grains, dried beans, low-fat dairy, and a variety of herbs and spices. Having these on hand makes it easier to prepare healthy meals without last-minute trips to the store.

✓ **Plan Your Meals:** Meal planning is key to maintaining a gout-friendly diet. Take some time each week to plan your meals and make a shopping list. This will help you stay on track and avoid unhealthy choices.

Equipping your kitchen with the right tools is an essential step in managing gout through diet. These tools not only make meal preparation easier and more enjoyable but also support your efforts to create healthy, delicious meals that are kind to your joints. With the right equipment and a well-organized kitchen, you'll be well on your way to taking control of your gout and living a healthier, more comfortable life.

2.2 Pantry Staples for Gout Management

Managing gout through diet involves making smart choices about the foods you keep in your kitchen. Stocking up on gout-friendly pantry staples ensures you always have the ingredients you need to prepare healthy, delicious meals that help control your uric acid levels and reduce the risk of painful flare-ups. Here's a comprehensive guide to the essential pantry staples for gout management.

Whole Grains

Whole grains are an excellent source of fiber and nutrients, and they can help you stay full and satisfied without increasing uric acid levels. Some gout-friendly whole grains to keep in your pantry include:

- ✓ **Brown Rice:** A versatile grain that can be used in a variety of dishes, from stir-fries to casseroles.

- ✓ **Quinoa:** A protein-rich grain that is great for salads, sides, and main dishes.

- ✓ **Oats:** Perfect for breakfast and baking, oats are a healthy and filling choice.

- ✓ **Whole Wheat Pasta:** A great alternative to refined pasta, providing more fiber and nutrients.

Legumes and Beans

Legumes and beans are excellent plant-based protein sources that are low in purines and high in fiber. They can be used in a variety of dishes, including soups, stews, salads, and casseroles. Keep a variety of dried and canned options on hand, such as:

- ✓ **Lentils:** Quick-cooking and versatile, lentils are perfect for soups, stews, and salads.

- ✓ **Chickpeas:** Great for making hummus, adding to salads, or roasting for a crunchy snack.

- ✓ **Black Beans:** Perfect for soups, stews, and Mexican-inspired dishes.

- ✓ **Kidney Beans:** A hearty addition to chilis and stews.

Low-fat Dairy Products

Low-fat dairy products have been shown to help lower uric acid levels and are an important part of a gout-friendly diet. Stock your pantry and fridge with:

- ✓ **Low-fat Milk:** A versatile ingredient for cooking and baking.

- ✓ **Low-fat Yogurt:** Great for breakfast, snacks, or as a base for smoothies.

- ✓ **Low-fat Cheese:** A tasty addition to salads, sandwiches, and main dishes.

Nuts and Seeds

Nuts and seeds provide healthy fats, protein, and fiber, making them a great snack or addition to meals. Keep a variety of unsalted options on hand, such as:

- ✓ **Almonds:** Perfect for snacking, adding to salads, or using in baking.

- ✓ **Walnuts:** Rich in omega-3 fatty acids, great for snacking or adding to oatmeal and salads.

- ✓ **Chia Seeds:** A nutritious addition to smoothies, yogurt, and baked goods.

- ✓ **Flaxseeds:** Can be added to smoothies, oatmeal, or used as an egg substitute in baking.

Healthy Fats and Oils

Healthy fats are important for overall health and can help reduce inflammation. Stock your pantry with:

- ✓ **Olive Oil:** A heart-healthy oil that is perfect for cooking and dressings.

- ✓ **Avocado Oil:** Great for high-heat cooking and dressings.

✓ **Canola Oil:** A versatile oil that is good for cooking and baking.

Fruits and Vegetables

Fruits and vegetables should be the cornerstone of a gout-friendly diet. While fresh produce is always best, it's also helpful to have some shelf-stable options on hand:

✓ **Canned Tomatoes:** A versatile ingredient for soups, stews, sauces, and casseroles.

✓ **Canned Vegetables:** Look for low-sodium options to use in soups, stews, and side dishes.

✓ **Dried Fruits:** Choose unsweetened varieties to add to oatmeal, yogurt, or as a snack.

✓ **Applesauce:** A healthy snack or baking ingredient.

Herbs and Spices

Herbs and spices add flavor to your meals without adding purines or extra calories. Stock your pantry with a variety of dried herbs and spices to keep your meals interesting and flavorful:

✓ **Basil, Oregano, and Thyme:** Great for Italian and Mediterranean dishes.

- ✓ **Cumin and Coriander:** Perfect for Mexican and Indian-inspired recipes.

- ✓ **Turmeric and Ginger:** Known for their anti-inflammatory properties.

- ✓ **Cinnamon and Nutmeg:** Great for baking and adding flavor to oatmeal and smoothies.

Hydration Essentials

Staying well-hydrated is crucial for managing gout. Keep these beverages in your pantry:

- ✓ **Water:** Always have plenty of water on hand. Consider keeping a pitcher of infused water in the fridge for variety.

- ✓ **Herbal Teas:** Many herbal teas are hydrating and some, like ginger or turmeric tea, have anti-inflammatory properties.

- ✓ **100% Fruit Juice:** While whole fruits are preferable, having small amounts of 100% fruit juice can be a good option for adding flavor to your water or as an occasional treat.

Snacks and Convenience Foods

Having healthy, gout-friendly snacks and convenience foods on hand can help you stay on track even when you're busy:

- ✓ **Rice Cakes:** A low-purine snack that can be topped with nut butter or avocado.

- ✓ **Whole Grain Crackers:** Pair with low-fat cheese or hummus for a satisfying snack.

- ✓ **Popcorn:** A whole grain snack that can be seasoned with your favorite herbs and spices.

Tips for Stocking Your Pantry

1. **Buy in Bulk:** For non-perishable items like whole grains, beans, and nuts, buying in bulk can save money and ensure you always have them on hand.

2. **Label and Organize:** Keep your pantry organized by labeling containers and arranging items by category. This makes it easier to find what you need and plan your meals.

3. **Rotate Stock:** Use the "first in, first out" method to ensure you're using older items before newer ones.

This helps reduce waste and keeps your pantry fresh.

4. **Plan Ahead:** Regularly review your pantry inventory and make a shopping list to replenish staples before you run out.

Stocking your pantry with these essential gout-friendly staples ensures you're always prepared to create healthy, delicious meals that support your efforts to manage gout. By keeping a well-organized pantry filled with nutritious options, you'll find it easier to stick to your dietary goals and enjoy a variety of satisfying meals. Remember, managing gout is a journey, and having the right ingredients at your fingertips is a crucial step toward better health and fewer flare-ups.

2.3 Tips for Meal Planning and Preparation

Meal planning and preparation are essential strategies for managing gout through diet. By taking a proactive approach to your meals, you can ensure that you're consuming a balanced diet that helps keep uric acid levels in check, reduces the risk of flare-ups, and supports overall health. Here are some practical tips to help you plan and prepare gout-friendly meals efficiently and effectively.

1. Plan Your Meals Weekly

Taking some time each week to plan your meals can make a significant difference in your diet. Here's how to get started:

- ✓ **Set Aside Time:** Dedicate a specific time each week for meal planning. Sunday afternoons or evenings often work well for many people.

- ✓ **Create a Menu:** Plan out your breakfast, lunch, dinner, and snacks for the week. Include a variety of foods to ensure you're getting a range of nutrients.

- ✓ **Consider Your Schedule:** Be realistic about your time and energy levels. Plan simpler meals for busier days and more elaborate dishes when you have more time to cook.

2. Make a Shopping List

A well-organized shopping list is crucial for efficient grocery shopping and avoiding impulse buys:

- ✓ **Categorize Your List:** Organize your list by sections of the grocery store (e.g., produce, dairy, grains) to make shopping quicker and more efficient.

✓ **Check Your Pantry:** Before you go shopping, check what you already have to avoid buying duplicates and reduce food waste.

✓ **Stick to the List:** Try to stick to your list to avoid purchasing items that may not align with your dietary goals.

3. Prep Ingredients in Advance

Preparing ingredients ahead of time can save you a lot of effort during busy weekdays:

✓ **Wash and Chop Vegetables:** Pre-wash and chop vegetables for the week and store them in airtight containers in the fridge. This makes it easier to throw together salads, stir-fries, or snacks.

✓ **Cook Grains and Legumes:** Batch-cook grains like brown rice or quinoa and legumes like lentils or chickpeas. Store them in the fridge or freezer for quick additions to meals.

✓ **Marinate Proteins:** Marinate lean meats or tofu ahead of time so they're ready to cook when you need them.

4. Batch Cooking and Freezing

Batch cooking is a fantastic way to ensure you always have healthy meals on hand:

✓ **Double Recipes:** When you cook, double the recipe and freeze half for later. This works well for soups, stews, casseroles, and chili.

✓ **Portion Out Meals:** Divide batch-cooked meals into individual portions before freezing. This makes it easy to grab a single serving when you need a quick meal.

✓ **Label and Date:** Clearly label and date your freezer containers so you can keep track of what you have and use older items first.

5. Use Leftovers Creatively

Leftovers don't have to be boring. Get creative and repurpose them into new meals:

✓ **Transform Leftovers:** Turn roasted vegetables into a frittata, add leftover chicken to a salad, or use cooked grains in a stir-fry.

✓ **Make a Soup:** Combine leftover vegetables, proteins, and grains with a low-sodium broth to create a quick and nutritious soup.

6. Healthy Snacks

Having healthy snacks on hand can help you avoid unhealthy choices and keep your energy levels stable throughout the day:

✓ **Pre-portion Snacks:** Divide snacks like nuts, seeds, and dried fruits into individual portions to grab when needed.

✓ **Keep Fresh Fruit Available:** Always have a bowl of fresh fruit on your counter for a quick and healthy snack.

✓ **Prepare Dips and Spreads:** Make batches of hummus, guacamole, or yogurt-based dips to enjoy with vegetables or whole grain crackers.

7. Stay Hydrated

Hydration is key in managing gout, so include beverages in your meal planning:

- ✓ **Infused Water:** Keep a pitcher of water infused with fruits, herbs, or cucumber in the fridge for a refreshing and hydrating drink.

- ✓ **Herbal Teas:** Stock up on a variety of herbal teas to enjoy hot or iced.

8. Be Flexible

While planning is important, it's also essential to stay flexible:

- ✓ **Adapt as Needed:** If you have leftovers, adjust your meal plan to incorporate them. If you find fresh produce on sale, adapt your recipes to include it.

- ✓ **Listen to Your Body:** Pay attention to your hunger and fullness cues, and adjust your portion sizes and meal timing as needed.

9. Focus on Balance

A gout-friendly diet should be balanced and varied:

- ✓ **Include a Variety of Foods:** Ensure each meal includes a mix of lean proteins, whole grains, and plenty of fruits and vegetables.

- ✓ **Watch Portions:** Keep an eye on portion sizes, especially for high-purine foods, to help manage uric acid levels.

Sample Weekly Meal Plan

To help you get started, here's a sample weekly meal plan for a gout-friendly diet:

Monday

- ✓ **Breakfast:** Overnight oats with berries and chia seeds.

- ✓ **Lunch:** Quinoa salad with chickpeas, cucumbers, tomatoes, and a lemon-tahini dressing.

- ✓ **Dinner:** Baked salmon with steamed broccoli and brown rice.

- ✓ **Snack:** Apple slices with almond butter.

Tuesday

- ✓ **Breakfast:** Smoothie with low-fat yogurt, spinach, banana, and berries.

- ✓ **Lunch:** Lentil soup with whole grain crackers.

- ✓ **Dinner:** Stir-fried tofu with mixed vegetables and soba noodles.

- ✓ **Snack:** Carrot sticks with hummus.

Wednesday

- ✓ **Breakfast:** Greek yogurt with honey, walnuts, and sliced strawberries.

- ✓ **Lunch:** Whole wheat pita with hummus, grilled chicken, and mixed greens.

- ✓ **Dinner:** Turkey chili with kidney beans and a side salad.

- ✓ **Snack:** Mixed nuts and dried fruit.

Thursday

- ✓ **Breakfast:** Scrambled eggs with spinach and whole grain toast.

- ✓ **Lunch:** Black bean and corn salad with avocado and lime dressing.

- ✓ **Dinner:** Baked cod with quinoa and roasted Brussels sprouts.

- ✓ **Snack:** Fresh fruit salad.

Friday

- ✓ **Breakfast:** Chia pudding with almond milk, honey, and blueberries.

- ✓ **Lunch:** Spinach and lentil salad with a balsamic vinaigrette.

- ✓ **Dinner:** Grilled chicken with brown rice and sautéed green beans.

- ✓ **Snack:** Rice cakes with avocado spread.

Saturday

- ✓ **Breakfast:** Whole grain waffles with fresh berries and a dollop of low-fat yogurt.

- ✓ **Lunch:** Chickpea and vegetable wrap with a side of mixed greens.

- ✓ **Dinner:** Vegetable curry with basmati rice and a cucumber salad.

- ✓ **Snack:** Pear slices with cottage cheese.

Sunday

- ✓ **Breakfast:** Smoothie bowl with granola, banana, and chia seeds.

- ✓ **Lunch:** Tomato and mozzarella salad with whole wheat baguette slices.

- ✓ **Dinner:** Baked eggplant Parmesan with a side of steamed spinach.

- ✓ **Snack:** Popcorn seasoned with nutritional yeast.

Effective meal planning and preparation are vital components of managing gout through diet. By organizing your meals, shopping smartly, and preparing ingredients in advance, you can ensure that you always have nutritious, gout-friendly options on hand. These strategies not only help manage your condition but also make it easier to enjoy a variety of delicious and satisfying meals. Remember, consistency is key, and with a bit of planning and preparation, you can take significant steps toward better health and fewer gout flare-ups.

CHAPTER THREE

UNDERSTANDING INGREDIENTS

3.1 Foods to Avoid

Navigating the world of food can be tricky, especially when managing a condition like gout. Knowing which foods to avoid is crucial to keeping flare-ups at bay and maintaining your health. This section will guide you through the foods that are best left off your plate if you're looking to manage gout effectively. Let's delve into the specifics of what to avoid and why these foods can be problematic for gout sufferers.

High-Purine Foods

Purines are substances found in many foods, and when your body breaks them down, it produces uric acid. For people with gout, high levels of uric acid can lead to painful flare-ups. Thus, it's essential to limit foods that are particularly high in purines.

- ✓ **Red Meat:** Beef, lamb, and pork are all high in purines. While occasional consumption might be okay, it's best to avoid these meats as much as possible. Opt for lean poultry or plant-based protein sources instead.

✓ **Organ Meats:** Liver, kidneys, and other organ meats are extremely high in purines and should be completely avoided. These foods can significantly spike uric acid levels.

✓ **Game Meats:** Meats like venison and wild game are also high in purines. They might be a rare treat for some, but they can be a trigger for gout flare-ups.

Certain Seafood

Seafood can be a healthy choice, but some types are high in purines and can exacerbate gout symptoms.

✓ **Shellfish:** Shrimp, crab, lobster, and other shellfish are high in purines. While delicious, they can be a significant trigger for gout.

✓ **Anchovies, Sardines, and Mackerel:** These oily fish are particularly high in purines and are best avoided.

✓ **Other High-Purine Fish:** Fish like tuna, trout, and haddock also fall into the high-purine category. Choose lower-purine fish like salmon or catfish instead.

GOUT DIET COOKBOOK

Sugary Foods and Beverages

Sugar, especially fructose, can increase uric acid production. Be mindful of your intake of sugary foods and drinks.

- ✓ **Soft Drinks and Sweetened Beverages:** Regular consumption of sugary sodas and fruit drinks can lead to increased uric acid levels. Stick to water, herbal teas, or other unsweetened beverages.

- ✓ **Candies and Sweets:** Processed sweets, including candies, cakes, and pastries, often contain high levels of sugar and can contribute to uric acid buildup.

- ✓ **Fruit Juices:** Even though they're natural, many fruit juices are high in fructose. Opt for whole fruits instead, which provide fiber and other nutrients that juice lacks.

Alcohol

Alcohol can be a major trigger for gout attacks, particularly certain types of alcohol.

- ✓ **Beer:** Beer is particularly high in purines and has been shown to significantly increase the risk of gout flare-ups.

- ✓ **Spirits:** While not as high in purines as beer, spirits like whiskey, vodka, and gin can still contribute to gout symptoms.

- ✓ **Wine:** Although wine is often considered a better choice, it can still affect uric acid levels and should be consumed in moderation, if at all.

Certain Vegetables and Legumes

While most vegetables are great for a gout-friendly diet, a few have moderate to high purine levels and should be eaten in moderation.

- ✓ **Asparagus:** This vegetable contains higher levels of purines compared to others. Enjoy it occasionally rather than frequently.

- ✓ **Spinach:** Another nutritious vegetable that is somewhat higher in purines. Balance its intake with other low-purine vegetables.

- ✓ **Mushrooms:** These can be moderately high in purines and should be eaten in limited amounts.

✓ **Legumes:** Foods like lentils, peas, and beans have moderate purine levels. They are healthy and can be included in a balanced diet but should be monitored if you notice they trigger your gout.

Processed and Refined Foods

Processed foods often contain hidden ingredients that can contribute to gout symptoms.

✓ **Processed Meats:** Hot dogs, sausages, and deli meats are not only high in purines but also contain additives and preservatives that aren't good for your overall health.

✓ **Refined Carbohydrates:** White bread, pasta, and white rice lack fiber and can lead to insulin resistance, which may increase uric acid levels. Opt for whole grain versions instead.

✓ **Snack Foods:** Chips, crackers, and other packaged snacks often contain unhealthy fats and added sugars. Choose whole, unprocessed foods for better health outcomes.

Understanding which foods to avoid is a critical step in managing gout through diet. By steering clear of high-purine foods, sugary beverages, certain types of alcohol, and overly processed items, you can significantly reduce your risk of painful flare-ups. Remember, the goal is not only to avoid gout triggers but also to embrace a balanced, nutritious diet that supports overall health and well-being. Making informed food choices will help you live more comfortably with gout and enjoy a higher quality of life.

3.2 Foods to Limit

While certain foods should be avoided to manage gout effectively, others can be consumed in moderation. These foods may have moderate purine levels or other properties that could contribute to gout flare-ups if eaten excessively. The key is to enjoy them sparingly and be mindful of portion sizes. Let's explore the foods you should limit in your diet to keep gout under control.

Moderate-Purine Foods

Moderate-purine foods can be part of a balanced diet but should be eaten in controlled amounts. These foods contribute to uric acid production, though not as significantly as high-purine foods.

- ✓ **Lean Meats:** Chicken and turkey are lower in purines compared to red meat but still contain moderate amounts. Stick to smaller portions and avoid eating them daily.

- ✓ **Certain Fish:** Salmon, catfish, and sole are lower in purines than other types of fish. Enjoy them occasionally and keep portion sizes reasonable.

- ✓ **Seafood:** Shrimp and crab are lower in purines than shellfish like oysters and mussels. Limit your intake to once or twice a week.

Dairy Products

Dairy products can be beneficial for gout management, but it's important to choose low-fat or fat-free options and consume them in moderation.

- ✓ **Low-Fat Milk:** Opt for skim or 1% milk. It can help lower uric acid levels, but be cautious of overconsumption if you're sensitive to dairy.

- ✓ **Low-Fat Yogurt:** A healthy choice that can be enjoyed daily, but keep an eye on added sugars in flavored varieties.

- ✓ **Cheese:** Choose low-fat cheeses and eat them in small amounts to avoid excess saturated fat, which can affect overall health.

Certain Vegetables

While vegetables are generally low in purines, some have higher levels and should be eaten in moderation.

- ✓ **Cauliflower:** A nutritious vegetable that can be enjoyed occasionally in controlled portions.

- ✓ **Green Peas:** These are higher in purines than other vegetables but can still be included in your diet in small amounts.

- ✓ **Spinach and Asparagus:** As mentioned earlier, these are healthy but should be limited due to their purine content.

Whole Grains and Legumes

Whole grains and legumes are important for a balanced diet, but some are moderately high in purines.

- ✓ **Whole Wheat Bread and Pasta:** Opt for whole grain varieties, which are better than refined grains but still contain moderate purines.

- ✓ **Oats:** Enjoy oats for their health benefits, but be mindful of portion sizes.

- ✓ **Legumes:** Beans, lentils, and peas are good plant-based protein sources but should be limited to moderate portions if you're sensitive to purines.

Alcohol

While some types of alcohol are best avoided entirely, others can be consumed in limited amounts.

- ✓ **Wine:** Moderate wine consumption may be less likely to trigger gout than beer or spirits. Limit intake to a glass or two per week, and avoid drinking during flare-ups.

- ✓ **Spirits:** If you choose to drink spirits, do so sparingly. Occasional consumption may be acceptable, but it's best to avoid making it a regular habit.

Sugary Foods and Beverages

Even though these should be avoided as much as possible, occasional indulgences in small quantities may be acceptable.

- ✓ **Fruit Juices:** Opt for whole fruits over fruit juices. If you do drink juice, limit it to a small glass and choose 100% juice without added sugars.

- ✓ **Sweetened Beverages:** Minimize consumption of sugary drinks like sodas and energy drinks. Reserve them for rare treats.

- ✓ **Desserts:** Enjoy sweets like cakes, cookies, and candies occasionally and in small portions to avoid spikes in uric acid levels.

Fatty and Fried Foods

Foods high in unhealthy fats can contribute to weight gain and overall inflammation, which may worsen gout symptoms.

- ✓ **Fried Foods:** Limit foods that are deep-fried or heavily battered. These are high in unhealthy fats and calories.

- ✓ **Fast Food:** Fast food is often high in unhealthy fats, salt, and calories. If you do indulge, choose healthier options like salads (with dressing on the side) or grilled items.

✓ **Saturated and Trans Fats:** Reduce intake of foods high in these fats, such as butter, margarine, and commercially baked goods.

Salty Foods

Excess salt can lead to water retention and increase the burden on your kidneys, affecting uric acid elimination.

✓ **Processed Foods:** Canned soups, frozen meals, and packaged snacks often contain high levels of salt. Opt for low-sodium versions when possible.

✓ **Condiments:** Use soy sauce, ketchup, and other salty condiments sparingly. Look for low-sodium alternatives to season your food.

Tips for Moderation

Managing the intake of these foods requires balance and mindfulness. Here are some tips to help you keep your diet gout-friendly:

✓ **Portion Control:** Pay attention to portion sizes to avoid overeating moderate-purine foods.

✓ **Variety:** Ensure your diet includes a wide variety of low-purine fruits, vegetables, and whole grains to get a broad range of nutrients.

✓ **Mindful Eating:** Practice mindful eating by paying attention to your hunger and fullness cues, and enjoy your food slowly to enhance satisfaction.

✓ **Meal Planning:** Incorporate these foods into your meal plan in a balanced way, ensuring they complement a diet rich in gout-friendly options.

✓ **Hydration:** Drink plenty of water to help your body flush out uric acid and stay hydrated, especially when consuming foods that need to be limited.

Limiting certain foods rather than eliminating them entirely can help you maintain a balanced, enjoyable diet while managing gout. By being mindful of your portions and making thoughtful choices, you can enjoy a variety of foods without compromising your health. Moderation is key to keeping uric acid levels in check and preventing painful gout flare-ups. Remember, a well-rounded diet, combined with other healthy lifestyle choices, can significantly improve your quality of life when living with gout.

3.3 Foods to Include

When managing gout through diet, focusing on foods that help lower uric acid levels and reduce inflammation is essential. Including these foods in your daily meals can support overall health and minimize the risk of painful flare-ups. Let's explore the nutritious foods that should be a regular part of your gout-friendly diet.

Low-Purine Foods

Opt for these low-purine foods to support your gout management efforts:

- ✓ **Fruits:** Enjoy a variety of fruits such as berries (strawberries, blueberries, raspberries), cherries, apples, oranges, and bananas. These are rich in vitamins, minerals, and antioxidants.

- ✓ **Vegetables:** Include plenty of leafy greens (spinach, kale, Swiss chard), cruciferous vegetables (broccoli, cauliflower, Brussels sprouts), and colorful vegetables like bell peppers, tomatoes, and carrots.

- ✓ **Whole Grains:** Choose whole grains such as brown rice, quinoa, oats, barley, and whole wheat bread and pasta. These provide fiber and essential nutrients.

✓ **Lean Proteins:** Opt for lean sources of protein like chicken, turkey, tofu, and legumes (lentils, chickpeas, black beans). These are lower in purines compared to red meats.

✓ **Dairy:** Include low-fat or fat-free dairy products like milk, yogurt, and cheese. These can help reduce uric acid levels.

✓ **Nuts and Seeds:** Enjoy unsalted nuts (almonds, walnuts) and seeds (chia seeds, flaxseeds) as snacks or additions to meals for healthy fats and protein.

✓ **Healthy Fats:** Incorporate sources of healthy fats such as olive oil, avocado, and fatty fish like salmon and trout. These fats have anti-inflammatory properties.

✓ **Herbs and Spices:** Flavor your meals with herbs like basil, oregano, cilantro, and spices such as turmeric, ginger, and garlic. These add taste without increasing purine levels.

Hydration

Proper hydration is crucial for managing gout. Drink plenty of water throughout the day to help flush out uric acid from your body. You can also enjoy herbal teas and incorporate water-rich foods like cucumbers and watermelon into your diet.

Cherries

Cherries, in particular, have been shown to have anti-inflammatory properties and may help reduce the frequency of gout attacks. Include fresh cherries or unsweetened cherry juice in your diet regularly.

Vitamin C-Rich Foods

Foods rich in vitamin C can help lower uric acid levels. Include citrus fruits (oranges, lemons), kiwi, strawberries, and bell peppers in your meals.

Coffee

Moderate coffee consumption has been associated with a lower risk of gout attacks. Enjoying a cup or two of coffee daily may help reduce uric acid levels and inflammation.

Plant-Based Proteins

Incorporating more plant-based proteins into your diet, such as tofu, tempeh, and legumes, can provide valuable nutrients and reduce the purine load compared to animal proteins.

Omega-3 Fatty Acids

Omega-3 fatty acids, found in fatty fish like salmon, trout, and sardines, as well as in flaxseeds and walnuts, have anti-inflammatory properties that can benefit gout management.

Fiber-Rich Foods

Fiber helps regulate digestion and can contribute to overall health. Include plenty of fiber-rich foods like fruits, vegetables, whole grains, and legumes in your meals.

Probiotic Foods

Probiotics, found in yogurt and fermented foods like sauerkraut and kimchi, can support gut health and potentially reduce inflammation associated with gout.

Tips for Incorporation

- ✓ **Meal Planning:** Plan your meals around these gout-friendly foods to ensure you're getting a balanced diet.

- ✓ **Variety:** Include a wide range of foods from different food groups to maximize nutrient intake.

- ✓ **Portion Control:** Pay attention to portion sizes, especially with higher-calorie foods like nuts and healthy fats.

- ✓ **Cooking Methods:** Choose healthy cooking methods like grilling, baking, steaming, or sautéing with minimal oil to retain nutrients.

- ✓ **Snack Smart:** Keep healthy snacks like fresh fruit, nuts, or yogurt on hand to curb cravings and maintain energy levels throughout the day.

- ✓ **Moderation:** While these foods are beneficial, moderation is key to maintaining a healthy balance and managing gout effectively.

By focusing on these nutritious foods and incorporating them into your daily meals, you can support your efforts to manage gout effectively. A well-rounded diet rich in fruits, vegetables, whole grains, lean proteins, and healthy fats not only helps control uric acid levels but also promotes overall health and well-being. Making informed food choices and maintaining a balanced diet are crucial steps toward living comfortably with gout and reducing the frequency and severity of flare-ups.

CHAPTER FOUR

BREAKFAST RECIPES

4.1 Smoothies and Juices

Breakfast is often hailed as the most important meal of the day, especially when you're managing gout. Starting your morning with nutritious, gout-friendly options can set the tone for the rest of your day. Smoothies and juices are excellent choices because they are not only delicious and refreshing but also allow you to pack in a variety of fruits, vegetables, and other healthy ingredients. Here are some delightful smoothie and juice recipes to kickstart your day on a healthy note.

Berry Blast Smoothie

Ingredients:

- ✓ 1 cup fresh or frozen mixed berries (strawberries, blueberries, raspberries)

- ✓ 1 ripe banana

- ✓ 1/2 cup low-fat yogurt or almond milk

- ✓ 1 tablespoon chia seeds or flaxseeds (optional)

- ✓ Honey or maple syrup to taste (optional)

✓ Ice cubes (if using fresh berries)

Instructions:

1. Place the berries, banana, yogurt or almond milk, and chia seeds or flaxseeds (if using) into a blender.

2. Blend until smooth and creamy.

3. Taste and adjust sweetness with honey or maple syrup, if desired.

4. Add ice cubes if using fresh berries and blend again until desired consistency is reached.

5. Pour into a glass and enjoy immediately.

Green Goddess Juice

Ingredients:

✓ 1 cucumber, peeled and chopped

✓ 1 green apple, cored and chopped

✓ 2 cups spinach or kale leaves

✓ 1/2 lemon, juiced

✓ 1-inch piece of fresh ginger, peeled

✓ 1-2 cups water or coconut water

✓ Ice cubes (optional)

Instructions:

1. In a juicer or high-speed blender, combine the cucumber, green apple, spinach or kale, lemon juice, and ginger.

2. Add water or coconut water to help blend, adjusting the amount based on your desired consistency.

3. Blend until smooth.

4. If using a blender, strain the mixture through a fine mesh sieve or nut milk bag to remove pulp, if desired.

5. Pour into a glass over ice cubes (if using) and serve immediately.

Tropical Sunshine Smoothie Bowl

Ingredients:

✓ 1 frozen banana, sliced

✓ 1/2 cup frozen mango chunks

✓ 1/2 cup pineapple chunks

✓ 1/2 cup coconut milk or almond milk

- ✓ Toppings: Fresh berries, sliced banana, shredded coconut, chia seeds, granola

Instructions:

1. In a blender, combine the frozen banana, mango chunks, pineapple chunks, and coconut or almond milk.

2. Blend until smooth and creamy, adding more liquid if needed to achieve desired consistency.

3. Pour the smoothie into a bowl.

4. Top with fresh berries, sliced banana, shredded coconut, chia seeds, and granola.

5. Enjoy with a spoon and savor the tropical flavors!

Protein-Packed Peanut Butter Smoothie

Ingredients:

- ✓ 1 ripe banana

- ✓ 1 tablespoon natural peanut butter

- ✓ 1/2 cup plain Greek yogurt

- ✓ 1/2 cup almond milk or dairy milk

- ✓ 1 tablespoon honey or maple syrup (optional)

✓ Ice cubes

Instructions:

1. In a blender, combine the banana, peanut butter, Greek yogurt, almond milk or dairy milk, and honey or maple syrup (if using).

2. Add ice cubes for a thicker consistency, if desired.

3. Blend until smooth and creamy.

4. Pour into a glass and enjoy this protein-packed smoothie to fuel your morning.

Tips for Enjoying Smoothies and Juices

✓ **Customize:** Feel free to adjust these recipes based on your taste preferences and dietary needs. Add more greens, reduce sweetness, or swap ingredients as desired.

✓ **Prep Ahead:** Prepare smoothie packs by portioning out ingredients in advance. Store them in the freezer for quick and easy breakfasts.

✓ **Balance:** Include a mix of fruits, vegetables, protein, and healthy fats in your smoothies and juices to create a well-rounded meal.

✓ **Stay Hydrated:** Smoothies and juices contribute to your daily hydration, especially important for managing gout.

These vibrant and nutritious smoothie and juice recipes are perfect additions to your gout-friendly breakfast repertoire. They not only provide essential nutrients and hydration but also taste delicious and can be customized to suit your preferences. Starting your day with a healthy breakfast sets a positive tone for your overall well-being, helping you manage gout effectively and enjoy a delicious start to each morning.

4.2 Low-Purine Breakfast Bowls

Creating satisfying and nutritious breakfast bowls that are low in purines can be both delicious and beneficial for managing gout. These bowls offer a combination of wholesome ingredients that provide essential nutrients while helping to maintain balanced uric acid levels. Here are some creative and flavorful low-purine breakfast bowl ideas to inspire your mornings.

1. Greek Yogurt and Berry Bowl

Ingredients:

- ✓ 1 cup plain Greek yogurt

- ✓ 1/2 cup fresh berries (such as strawberries, blueberries, raspberries)

- ✓ 1/4 cup nuts (almonds, walnuts) or seeds (chia seeds, flaxseeds)

- ✓ 1 tablespoon honey or maple syrup (optional)

- ✓ Granola or whole grain cereal (optional)

Instructions:

1. Spoon Greek yogurt into a bowl.

2. Top with fresh berries and nuts or seeds.

3. Drizzle with honey or maple syrup, if desired.

4. Sprinkle with granola or whole grain cereal for added crunch.

5. Enjoy this protein-rich and antioxidant-packed breakfast bowl.

2. Quinoa and Vegetable Breakfast Bowl

Ingredients:

- ✓ 1/2 cup cooked quinoa

- ✓ 1/2 cup sautéed spinach or kale

- ✓ 1/4 cup diced cucumber

- ✓ 1/4 cup diced bell peppers (any color)

- ✓ 1/4 cup cherry tomatoes, halved

- ✓ 1 tablespoon olive oil

- ✓ Fresh lemon juice, to taste

- ✓ Salt and pepper, to taste

- ✓ Optional: Poached or boiled egg for added protein

Instructions:

1. In a bowl, layer cooked quinoa and sautéed spinach or kale.

2. Add diced cucumber, bell peppers, and cherry tomatoes.

3. Drizzle with olive oil and fresh lemon juice.

4. Season with salt and pepper to taste.

5. Top with a poached or boiled egg, if desired, for extra protein and richness.

6. Enjoy this nutritious and satisfying breakfast bowl.

3. Avocado and Egg Breakfast Bowl

Ingredients:

- ✓ 1 ripe avocado, sliced or mashed

- ✓ 2 boiled or poached eggs, sliced

- ✓ 1/2 cup diced tomatoes

- ✓ 1/4 cup diced red onion

- ✓ Fresh cilantro or parsley, chopped

- ✓ Salt and pepper, to taste

- ✓ Optional: Sprinkle of feta cheese or a drizzle of balsamic glaze

Instructions:

1. Arrange sliced or mashed avocado in a bowl.

2. Top with sliced boiled or poached eggs.

3. Add diced tomatoes and red onion.

4. Sprinkle with chopped cilantro or parsley.

5. Season with salt and pepper to taste.

6. Optional: Add a sprinkle of feta cheese or a drizzle of balsamic glaze for extra flavor.

7. Enjoy this creamy, protein-packed breakfast bowl.

4. Chia Seed Pudding Bowl

Ingredients:

- ✓ 1/4 cup chia seeds

- ✓ 1 cup almond milk or coconut milk

- ✓ 1/2 teaspoon vanilla extract

- ✓ Fresh berries or sliced fruits

- ✓ Nuts or seeds (optional for topping)

- ✓ Honey or maple syrup (optional for sweetness)

Instructions:

1. In a bowl or jar, combine chia seeds, almond milk or coconut milk, and vanilla extract.

2. Stir well to combine, ensuring all chia seeds are submerged in liquid.

3. Refrigerate for at least 2 hours or overnight, stirring occasionally, until mixture thickens into a pudding-like consistency.

4. Spoon chia seed pudding into a bowl.

5. Top with fresh berries or sliced fruits and nuts or seeds, if using.

6. Drizzle with honey or maple syrup for added sweetness, if desired.

7. Enjoy this fiber-rich and nutrient-dense breakfast bowl.

Tips for Low-Purine Breakfast Bowls

✓ **Variety:** Experiment with different combinations of grains, vegetables, fruits, and proteins to keep your breakfast bowls interesting and nutritious.

✓ **Preparation:** Cook grains like quinoa or prepare chia seed pudding ahead of time for quick assembly in the morning.

- ✓ **Balance:** Include a mix of textures and flavors to create satisfying breakfast bowls that keep you full and energized.

- ✓ **Portion Control:** Be mindful of portion sizes, especially when adding nuts, seeds, or toppings like granola.

- ✓ **Customization:** Adapt recipes to suit your taste preferences and dietary needs, such as adding more vegetables or adjusting seasoning.

These low-purine breakfast bowl recipes offer delicious and nourishing options to support your gout management efforts. Packed with wholesome ingredients and customizable to your liking, they provide a satisfying start to your day while helping to maintain balanced uric acid levels. Enjoy these nutritious breakfast bowls as part of a well-rounded diet that promotes overall health and well-being.

4.3 Healthy Breakfast Ideas

Starting your day with a nutritious breakfast is essential for overall health and well-being, especially when managing conditions like gout. These healthy breakfast ideas are packed with essential nutrients, low in purines, and delicious enough to kickstart your day on a positive note.

1. Overnight Oats with Fresh Fruits

Ingredients:

- ✓ 1/2 cup rolled oats

- ✓ 1/2 cup almond milk or dairy milk

- ✓ 1/4 cup Greek yogurt

- ✓ 1 tablespoon chia seeds

- ✓ 1/2 teaspoon vanilla extract

- ✓ Fresh fruits (such as berries, sliced banana)

- ✓ Optional toppings: Nuts (almonds, walnuts), seeds (sunflower seeds), honey or maple syrup

Instructions:

1. In a jar or bowl, combine rolled oats, almond milk or dairy milk, Greek yogurt, chia seeds, and vanilla extract.

2. Stir well to mix all ingredients thoroughly.

3. Cover the jar or bowl and refrigerate overnight, or for at least 4 hours, to allow oats to soften and absorb liquid.

4. In the morning, stir the overnight oats mixture and top with fresh fruits, nuts, seeds, and a drizzle of honey or maple syrup if desired.

5. Enjoy this creamy and nutrient-packed breakfast bowl cold or at room temperature.

2. Veggie Omelette with Whole Grain Toast

Ingredients:

- ✓ 2 large eggs
- ✓ 1/4 cup diced bell peppers (any color)
- ✓ 1/4 cup diced tomatoes
- ✓ 1/4 cup chopped spinach or kale
- ✓ Salt and pepper, to taste
- ✓ 1 teaspoon olive oil or cooking spray
- ✓ 1 slice whole grain toast

Instructions:

1. In a bowl, whisk together eggs, diced bell peppers, tomatoes, chopped spinach or kale, salt, and pepper.

2. Heat olive oil or cooking spray in a non-stick skillet over medium heat.

3. Pour egg mixture into the skillet and cook for 2-3 minutes, lifting edges with a spatula to allow uncooked egg to flow underneath.

4. Once the omelette is set, fold it in half and cook for another 1-2 minutes until fully cooked through.

5. Serve the veggie omelette with a slice of whole grain toast on the side.

6. Enjoy this protein-rich and fiber-packed breakfast that keeps you satisfied until lunchtime.

3. Quinoa Breakfast Bowl with Avocado and Poached Egg

Ingredients:

- ✓ 1/2 cup cooked quinoa

- ✓ 1/4 avocado, sliced

- ✓ 1 poached or boiled egg

- ✓ 1/4 cup cherry tomatoes, halved

- ✓ Fresh herbs (cilantro, parsley), chopped

- ✓ Salt and pepper, to taste

Instructions:

1. In a bowl, layer cooked quinoa, sliced avocado, poached or boiled egg, and cherry tomatoes.

2. Sprinkle with chopped fresh herbs, salt, and pepper.

3. Enjoy this protein-packed and nutrient-dense breakfast bowl that's bursting with flavors and textures.

4. Smoothie Bowl with Nut Butter and Granola

Ingredients:

- ✓ 1 frozen banana

- ✓ 1/2 cup frozen berries (such as strawberries, blueberries)

- ✓ 1/4 cup almond milk or dairy milk

- ✓ 1 tablespoon nut butter (peanut butter, almond butter)

- ✓ Toppings: Granola, sliced banana, nuts (almonds, walnuts), seeds (chia seeds)

Instructions:

1. In a blender, combine frozen banana, frozen berries, almond milk or dairy milk, and nut butter.

2. Blend until smooth and creamy, adding more liquid if needed to achieve desired consistency.

3. Pour the smoothie into a bowl.

4. Top with granola, sliced banana, nuts, and seeds.

5. Enjoy this refreshing and energy-boosting smoothie bowl for a nutritious breakfast option.

Tips for Healthy Breakfast Ideas

- ✓ **Balance:** Include a mix of protein, fiber, healthy fats, and carbohydrates in your breakfast to keep you full and satisfied.

- ✓ **Variety:** Rotate your breakfast options to ensure you get a wide range of nutrients and flavors.

- ✓ **Preparation:** Prep ingredients ahead of time for quick assembly in the morning, such as cooking quinoa or chopping vegetables.

- ✓ **Hydration:** Pair your breakfast with water, herbal tea, or a glass of fruit-infused water to stay hydrated throughout the day.

These healthy breakfast ideas are designed to support your gout management goals while providing delicious and nutritious options to start your day. Whether you prefer overnight oats, veggie omelettes, quinoa bowls, or smoothie bowls, each recipe offers a balance of essential nutrients and flavors to keep you energized and satisfied. Enjoy these breakfasts as part of a well-rounded diet that promotes overall health and well-being.

CHAPTER FIVE

LUNCH RECIPES

5.1 Fresh Salads and Dressings

Lunchtime offers a perfect opportunity to refuel your body with nutrient-dense foods that support your gout management journey. Fresh salads with vibrant vegetables, lean proteins, and flavorful dressings not only satisfy your hunger but also contribute to overall well-being. Here are some delicious and gout-friendly salad recipes along with homemade dressings to elevate your midday meal.

1. Classic Garden Salad

Ingredients:

- ✓ Mixed salad greens (lettuce, spinach, arugula)
- ✓ Cherry tomatoes, halved
- ✓ Cucumber, sliced
- ✓ Carrot, shredded
- ✓ Red onion, thinly sliced
- ✓ Optional additions: Bell peppers, radishes, avocado slices

Instructions:

1. In a large bowl, combine mixed salad greens, cherry tomatoes, cucumber, carrot, red onion, and any optional additions you like.

2. Toss gently to mix ingredients evenly.

3. Serve with your choice of homemade dressing (see dressing recipes below) or a drizzle of olive oil and balsamic vinegar.

2. Grilled Chicken Caesar Salad

Ingredients:

- ✓ Grilled chicken breast, sliced
- ✓ Romaine lettuce, chopped
- ✓ Croutons (optional)
- ✓ Parmesan cheese, shaved or grated
- ✓ Caesar dressing (homemade recipe below)

Instructions:

1. Arrange chopped romaine lettuce on a plate.

2. Top with sliced grilled chicken breast, croutons (if using), and shaved or grated Parmesan cheese.

3. Drizzle with Caesar dressing and toss gently to coat.

4. Enjoy this protein-packed and satisfying salad.

3. Quinoa and Vegetable Salad

Ingredients:

- ✓ 1/2 cup cooked quinoa

- ✓ Mixed vegetables (bell peppers, cherry tomatoes, cucumber, red onion)

- ✓ Fresh herbs (parsley, basil), chopped

- ✓ Lemon vinaigrette dressing (homemade recipe below)

Instructions:

1. In a bowl, combine cooked quinoa, mixed vegetables, and chopped fresh herbs.

2. Drizzle with lemon vinaigrette dressing and toss gently to combine.

3. Serve chilled or at room temperature as a refreshing and nutritious salad option.

4. Homemade Dressing Recipes

1. Lemon Vinaigrette

Ingredients:

- ✓ 1/4 cup fresh lemon juice
- ✓ 1/2 cup olive oil
- ✓ 1 garlic clove, minced
- ✓ 1 teaspoon Dijon mustard
- ✓ 1 teaspoon honey or maple syrup
- ✓ Salt and pepper, to taste

Instructions:

1. In a small bowl or jar, whisk together lemon juice, olive oil, minced garlic, Dijon mustard, honey or maple syrup, salt, and pepper until well combined.

2. Adjust seasoning to taste.

3. Store any leftover dressing in a sealed container in the refrigerator for up to one week.

5. Caesar Dressing

Ingredients:

- ✓ 1/2 cup mayonnaise or Greek yogurt
- ✓ 2 tablespoons grated Parmesan cheese
- ✓ 1 tablespoon fresh lemon juice
- ✓ 1 garlic clove, minced
- ✓ 1 teaspoon Dijon mustard
- ✓ Salt and pepper, to taste

Instructions:

1. In a bowl, whisk together mayonnaise or Greek yogurt, grated Parmesan cheese, lemon juice, minced garlic, Dijon mustard, salt, and pepper until smooth and creamy.

2. Adjust seasoning to taste.

3. Refrigerate in a sealed container until ready to use.

Tips for Enjoying Fresh Salads

- ✓ **Prep Ahead:** Wash and chop salad ingredients in advance for quick assembly during busy days.

- ✓ **Protein Boost:** Add grilled chicken, shrimp, tofu, or beans to salads to increase protein content and make them more satisfying.

- ✓ **Variety:** Experiment with different combinations of vegetables, fruits, nuts, and seeds to keep your salads interesting and nutritious.

- ✓ **Portion Control:** Be mindful of portion sizes for toppings and dressings to maintain a balanced meal.

These fresh salad recipes and homemade dressings provide delicious options for a gout-friendly lunch that's both nutritious and satisfying. Whether you prefer a classic garden salad, a protein-packed Caesar salad, or a quinoa and vegetable salad, each recipe is designed to support your health goals while offering vibrant flavors and textures. Enjoy these salads as part of a well-rounded diet that promotes overall well-being and helps manage gout effectively.

5.2 Gout-Friendly Sandwiches and Wraps

Sandwiches and wraps are convenient and versatile options for a satisfying lunch that can be tailored to fit a gout-friendly diet. By choosing wholesome ingredients and flavorful combinations, you can enjoy delicious meals that support your health goals. Here are some tasty and nutritious sandwich and wrap recipes to inspire your next lunch.

1. Grilled Chicken and Avocado Wrap

Ingredients:

- ✓ Whole grain wrap or tortilla
- ✓ Grilled chicken breast, sliced
- ✓ 1/4 avocado, sliced
- ✓ Mixed salad greens (lettuce, spinach)
- ✓ Tomato slices
- ✓ Optional: Thinly sliced red onion, hummus

Instructions:

1. Lay the whole grain wrap or tortilla flat on a clean surface.

2. Layer grilled chicken breast slices, avocado slices, mixed salad greens, tomato slices, and any optional additions you like (such as red onion or hummus) evenly across the wrap.

3. Roll the wrap tightly, folding in the sides as you go.

4. Slice in half diagonally and secure with toothpicks if needed.

5. Enjoy this protein-rich and flavorful wrap for a satisfying lunch.

2. Mediterranean Veggie Sandwich

Ingredients:

- ✓ Whole grain bread slices

- ✓ Hummus

- ✓ Sliced cucumber

- ✓ Sliced bell peppers (any color)

- ✓ Sliced tomatoes

- ✓ Red onion, thinly sliced

- ✓ Fresh basil leaves

- ✓ Feta cheese, crumbled (optional)

Instructions:

1. Spread hummus evenly on whole grain bread slices.

2. Layer sliced cucumber, bell peppers, tomatoes, red onion, fresh basil leaves, and crumbled feta cheese (if using) on one slice of bread.

3. Top with the other bread slice and press gently to pack ingredients together.

4. Slice the sandwich in half and serve immediately.

5. Enjoy this Mediterranean-inspired sandwich filled with fresh flavors and nutrients.

3. Tuna Salad Lettuce Wraps

Ingredients:

- ✓ Canned tuna, drained
- ✓ Greek yogurt or mayonnaise
- ✓ Diced celery
- ✓ Diced red onion
- ✓ Fresh lemon juice
- ✓ Salt and pepper, to taste
- ✓ Lettuce leaves (such as romaine or butter lettuce)

Instructions:

1. In a bowl, mix canned tuna, Greek yogurt or mayonnaise, diced celery, diced red onion, fresh lemon juice, salt, and pepper until well combined.

2. Spoon tuna salad mixture onto lettuce leaves.

3. Roll up the lettuce leaves to create wraps.

4. Secure with toothpicks if needed.

5. Enjoy these light and flavorful tuna salad lettuce wraps for a protein-packed lunch option.

4. Caprese Panini

Ingredients:

- ✓ Whole grain bread slices

- ✓ Fresh mozzarella cheese, sliced

- ✓ Tomato slices

- ✓ Fresh basil leaves

- ✓ Balsamic glaze or reduction

- ✓ Olive oil or cooking spray

Instructions:

1. Layer fresh mozzarella cheese slices, tomato slices, and fresh basil leaves between two slices of whole grain bread.

2. Drizzle with balsamic glaze or reduction.

3. Heat a panini press or skillet over medium heat and lightly coat with olive oil or cooking spray.

4. Place the assembled sandwich in the panini press or skillet and cook until the bread is golden brown and the cheese is melted.

5. Slice the panini in half diagonally and serve hot.

6. Enjoy this classic Caprese panini filled with Italian flavors.

Tips for Gout-Friendly Sandwiches and Wraps

✓ **Whole Grains:** Opt for whole grain breads or wraps to increase fiber content and promote satiety.

✓ **Lean Proteins:** Choose lean protein sources such as grilled chicken, tuna, or hummus to reduce purine intake.

- ✓ **Fresh Vegetables:** Load sandwiches and wraps with colorful vegetables for added vitamins, minerals, and antioxidants.

- ✓ **Portion Control:** Be mindful of portion sizes, especially with condiments and cheeses, to maintain a balanced meal.

These gout-friendly sandwich and wrap recipes offer delicious and nutritious options for a satisfying lunch. Whether you prefer a grilled chicken and avocado wrap, a Mediterranean veggie sandwich, tuna salad lettuce wraps, or a Caprese panini, each recipe is designed to support your health goals while providing flavorful combinations that you'll enjoy. Incorporate these meals into your weekly lunch rotation for a well-rounded diet that promotes overall well-being and helps manage gout effectively.

5.3 Hearty Soups and Stews

Soups and stews are comforting and nourishing options for a hearty lunch that can be adapted to fit a gout-friendly diet. Packed with wholesome ingredients, these recipes provide warmth and satisfaction while supporting your health goals.

Here are some flavorful and nutritious soup and stew recipes to elevate your lunchtime experience.

1. Lentil and Vegetable Soup

Ingredients:

- ✓ 1 cup dried lentils, rinsed
- ✓ 4 cups vegetable broth or water
- ✓ 1 onion, diced
- ✓ 2 carrots, diced
- ✓ 2 celery stalks, diced
- ✓ 2 garlic cloves, minced
- ✓ 1 teaspoon dried thyme
- ✓ 1 teaspoon dried rosemary
- ✓ Salt and pepper, to taste
- ✓ Fresh parsley, chopped (for garnish)
- ✓ Lemon wedges (optional)

Instructions:

1. In a large pot, heat olive oil over medium heat.

2. Add diced onion, carrots, and celery. Sauté until vegetables are softened, about 5-7 minutes.

3. Add minced garlic, dried thyme, and dried rosemary. Sauté for another 1-2 minutes until fragrant.

4. Add rinsed lentils and vegetable broth or water to the pot. Bring to a boil.

5. Reduce heat to low, cover, and simmer for 20-25 minutes or until lentils are tender.

6. Season with salt and pepper to taste.

7. Ladle soup into bowls and garnish with chopped fresh parsley.

8. Serve with lemon wedges on the side for added brightness, if desired.

9. Enjoy this hearty and nutritious lentil and vegetable soup.

2. Chicken and Vegetable Stew

Ingredients:

- ✓ 1 tablespoon olive oil

- ✓ 1 onion, diced

- ✓ 2 garlic cloves, minced

- ✓ 2 carrots, sliced

- ✓ 2 celery stalks, sliced

- ✓ 1 bell pepper, diced

- ✓ 1 zucchini, diced

- ✓ 1 pound chicken breast or thigh, diced

- ✓ 4 cups chicken broth

- ✓ 1 teaspoon dried thyme

- ✓ 1 teaspoon dried oregano

- ✓ Salt and pepper, to taste

- ✓ Fresh parsley, chopped (for garnish)

Instructions:

1. In a large pot or Dutch oven, heat olive oil over medium heat.

2. Add diced onion and minced garlic. Sauté until onion is translucent, about 3-4 minutes.

3. Add sliced carrots, celery, bell pepper, and zucchini. Sauté for another 5 minutes until vegetables begin to soften.

4. Add diced chicken to the pot. Cook until chicken is browned on all sides, about 5-7 minutes.

5. Pour in chicken broth and stir in dried thyme and oregano.

6. Bring stew to a boil, then reduce heat to low. Cover and simmer for 20-25 minutes or until chicken is cooked through and vegetables are tender.

7. Season with salt and pepper to taste.

8. Ladle stew into bowls and garnish with chopped fresh parsley.

9. Enjoy this comforting and protein-rich chicken and vegetable stew.

3. Tomato Basil Soup

Ingredients:

- ✓ 2 tablespoons olive oil

- ✓ 1 onion, diced

- ✓ 2 garlic cloves, minced

- ✓ 1 can (28 ounces) crushed tomatoes

- ✓ 2 cups vegetable broth

- ✓ 1 teaspoon dried basil

- ✓ 1/2 teaspoon dried oregano

- ✓ Salt and pepper, to taste

- ✓ Fresh basil leaves, chopped (for garnish)

- ✓ Optional: Heavy cream or coconut milk (for creamier texture)

Instructions:

1. In a large pot, heat olive oil over medium heat.

2. Add diced onion and minced garlic. Sauté until onion is translucent, about 3-4 minutes.

3. Add crushed tomatoes, vegetable broth, dried basil, and dried oregano to the pot. Stir to combine.

4. Bring soup to a boil, then reduce heat to low. Cover and simmer for 15-20 minutes to allow flavors to meld.

5. If desired, stir in heavy cream or coconut milk for a creamier texture.

6. Season with salt and pepper to taste.

7. Ladle soup into bowls and garnish with chopped fresh basil leaves.

8. Enjoy this classic tomato basil soup as a comforting and flavorful lunch option.

Tips for Enjoying Hearty Soups and Stews

- ✓ **Batch Cooking:** Prepare soups and stews in large batches and store leftovers in the refrigerator or freezer for quick and easy meals throughout the week.

- ✓ **Whole Grains:** Serve soups and stews with whole grain bread or brown rice for added fiber and nutrients.

- ✓ **Vegetable Variety:** Experiment with different vegetables and herbs to customize flavors and boost nutritional content.

- ✓ **Slow Cooking:** Use a slow cooker or crockpot for hands-off cooking and tender results.

✓ **Hydration:** Enjoy soups and stews with a glass of water or herbal tea to stay hydrated.

These hearty soup and stew recipes offer nourishing and flavorful options for a gout-friendly lunch. Whether you prefer a comforting lentil and vegetable soup, a protein-rich chicken and vegetable stew, or a classic tomato basil soup, each recipe is designed to support your health goals while providing warmth and satisfaction. Incorporate these meals into your weekly lunch rotation for a delicious and nutritious way to manage gout effectively and promote overall well-being.

CHAPTER SIX

DINNER RECIPES

6.1 Low-Purine Main Dishes

Dinner is a time to unwind and nourish your body with delicious and nutritious meals that support your gout management goals. Choosing low-purine main dishes allows you to enjoy flavorful dinners while maintaining balanced uric acid levels. Here are some satisfying and gout-friendly main dish recipes to elevate your evening meals.

1. Grilled Salmon with Quinoa and Roasted Vegetables

Ingredients:

- ✓ 4 salmon fillets
- ✓ 1 cup quinoa, rinsed
- ✓ 2 cups water or vegetable broth
- ✓ 1 red bell pepper, sliced
- ✓ 1 zucchini, sliced
- ✓ 1 yellow squash, sliced
- ✓ 1 red onion, sliced

- ✓ 2 tablespoons olive oil

- ✓ 1 teaspoon dried thyme

- ✓ Salt and pepper, to taste

- ✓ Fresh lemon wedges (for serving)

Instructions:

1. Preheat oven to 400°F (200°C).

2. In a saucepan, bring water or vegetable broth to a boil. Add rinsed quinoa, cover, and simmer for 15-20 minutes or until quinoa is cooked and liquid is absorbed.

3. Meanwhile, toss sliced red bell pepper, zucchini, yellow squash, and red onion with olive oil, dried thyme, salt, and pepper on a baking sheet.

4. Roast vegetables in the preheated oven for 20-25 minutes, stirring halfway through, until tender and lightly browned.

5. Season salmon fillets with salt and pepper. Grill salmon over medium-high heat for 4-5 minutes per side, or until fish flakes easily with a fork.

6. Serve grilled salmon alongside cooked quinoa and roasted vegetables.

7. Squeeze fresh lemon juice over salmon before serving for added brightness.

8. Enjoy this protein-packed and nutrient-dense dinner.

2. Turkey and Vegetable Stir-Fry

Ingredients:

- ✓ 1 pound turkey breast, sliced

- ✓ 2 tablespoons low-sodium soy sauce

- ✓ 1 tablespoon rice vinegar

- ✓ 1 tablespoon honey or maple syrup

- ✓ 2 tablespoons olive oil

- ✓ 1 onion, thinly sliced

- ✓ 2 bell peppers (any color), sliced

- ✓ 1 cup snow peas

- ✓ 1 carrot, sliced

- ✓ 2 garlic cloves, minced

- ✓ Cooked brown rice or quinoa (for serving)

- ✓ Fresh cilantro or green onions, chopped (for garnish)

Instructions:

1. In a bowl, whisk together low-sodium soy sauce, rice vinegar, and honey or maple syrup. Set aside.

2. Heat olive oil in a large skillet or wok over medium-high heat.

3. Add sliced turkey breast and stir-fry for 5-7 minutes until browned and cooked through. Remove from skillet and set aside.

4. In the same skillet, add more olive oil if needed. Add thinly sliced onion, bell peppers, snow peas, carrot, and minced garlic. Stir-fry for 3-4 minutes until vegetables are tender-crisp.

5. Return cooked turkey breast to the skillet. Pour in the soy sauce mixture and toss everything together to coat evenly.

6. Cook for another 1-2 minutes until heated through and flavors are combined.

7. Serve turkey and vegetable stir-fry over cooked brown rice or quinoa.

8. Garnish with chopped fresh cilantro or green onions.

9. Enjoy this colorful and flavorful turkey and vegetable stir-fry for a satisfying dinner.

3. Eggplant and Chickpea Curry

Ingredients:

- ✓ 1 large eggplant, diced
- ✓ 1 can (15 ounces) chickpeas, drained and rinsed
- ✓ 1 onion, diced
- ✓ 2 garlic cloves, minced
- ✓ 1 tablespoon grated ginger
- ✓ 1 can (14 ounces) diced tomatoes
- ✓ 1 can (14 ounces) coconut milk
- ✓ 1 tablespoon curry powder
- ✓ 1 teaspoon ground cumin

- ✓ 1/2 teaspoon ground turmeric

- ✓ Salt and pepper, to taste

- ✓ Fresh cilantro, chopped (for garnish)

- ✓ Cooked brown rice or quinoa (for serving)

Instructions:

1. Heat olive oil in a large pot or Dutch oven over medium heat.

2. Add diced onion and cook until translucent, about 3-4 minutes.

3. Add minced garlic and grated ginger. Cook for another 1-2 minutes until fragrant.

4. Stir in diced eggplant, chickpeas, diced tomatoes, coconut milk, curry powder, ground cumin, and ground turmeric.

5. Season with salt and pepper to taste.

6. Bring curry to a boil, then reduce heat to low. Cover and simmer for 20-25 minutes, stirring occasionally, until eggplant is tender.

7. Serve eggplant and chickpea curry over cooked brown rice or quinoa.

8. Garnish with chopped fresh cilantro.

9. Enjoy this aromatic and satisfying eggplant and chickpea curry for a flavorful dinner.

Tips for Low-Purine Main Dishes

✓ **Lean Proteins:** Choose lean meats like turkey, chicken, and fish over high-purine options.

✓ **Plant-Based Proteins:** Incorporate legumes such as chickpeas and lentils for protein without the purines found in meat.

✓ **Colorful Vegetables:** Include a variety of colorful vegetables to boost nutritional content and add vibrant flavors.

✓ **Whole Grains:** Serve main dishes with whole grains like quinoa or brown rice for added fiber and nutrients.

✓ **Herbs and Spices:** Use herbs and spices generously to enhance flavors without relying on high-sodium seasonings.

These low-purine main dish recipes offer flavorful and satisfying options for a gout-friendly dinner. Whether you prefer grilled salmon with quinoa and roasted vegetables, turkey and vegetable stir-fry, or eggplant and chickpea curry, each recipe is designed to support your health goals while providing delicious meals that you'll enjoy. Incorporate these dishes into your weekly dinner rotation for a balanced diet that promotes overall well-being and helps manage gout effectively.

6.2 Vegetable-Forward Entrees

Embracing vegetable-forward entrees not only supports a gout-friendly diet but also brings a burst of flavors and nutrients to your dinner table. These recipes highlight the natural goodness of vegetables while offering satisfying and wholesome meals. Here are some delicious and nutritious vegetable-forward entrees to inspire your evening meals.

1. Stuffed Bell Peppers with Quinoa and Black Beans

Ingredients:

- ✓ 4 bell peppers (any color)
- ✓ 1 cup quinoa, rinsed
- ✓ 2 cups vegetable broth or water

- ✓ 1 can (15 ounces) black beans, drained and rinsed

- ✓ 1 cup corn kernels (fresh or frozen)

- ✓ 1 onion, diced

- ✓ 2 garlic cloves, minced

- ✓ 1 teaspoon ground cumin

- ✓ 1 teaspoon chili powder

- ✓ Salt and pepper, to taste

- ✓ Fresh cilantro, chopped (for garnish)

- ✓ Optional: Shredded cheese (such as cheddar or Monterey Jack)

Instructions:

1. Preheat oven to 375°F (190°C).

2. Cut the tops off bell peppers and remove seeds and membranes.

3. In a saucepan, bring vegetable broth or water to a boil. Add rinsed quinoa, cover, and simmer for 15-20 minutes or until quinoa is cooked and liquid is absorbed.

4. Meanwhile, heat olive oil in a skillet over medium heat. Add diced onion and cook until translucent, about 3-4 minutes.

5. Add minced garlic, ground cumin, and chili powder. Cook for another 1-2 minutes until fragrant.

6. Stir in black beans and corn kernels. Cook for 3-4 minutes until heated through.

7. Remove skillet from heat and stir in cooked quinoa. Season with salt and pepper to taste.

8. Stuff bell peppers with quinoa and black bean mixture.

9. Place stuffed bell peppers in a baking dish. If desired, sprinkle shredded cheese on top.

10. Bake in the preheated oven for 25-30 minutes or until bell peppers are tender and cheese is melted.

11. Garnish with chopped fresh cilantro before serving.

12. Enjoy these colorful and nutritious stuffed bell peppers as a satisfying vegetable-forward entree.

2. Ratatouille

GOUT DIET COOKBOOK

Ingredients:

- ✓ 1 eggplant, diced
- ✓ 2 zucchinis, diced
- ✓ 1 yellow squash, diced
- ✓ 1 onion, diced
- ✓ 2 bell peppers (any color), diced
- ✓ 2 garlic cloves, minced
- ✓ 2 cups diced tomatoes (fresh or canned)
- ✓ 1 tablespoon tomato paste
- ✓ 1 teaspoon dried thyme
- ✓ 1 teaspoon dried oregano
- ✓ Salt and pepper, to taste
- ✓ Fresh basil leaves, chopped (for garnish)
- ✓ Optional: Grated Parmesan cheese

Instructions:

1. Heat olive oil in a large skillet or Dutch oven over medium heat.

2. Add diced eggplant, zucchinis, yellow squash, onion, and bell peppers to the skillet. Cook for 8-10 minutes, stirring occasionally, until vegetables are softened.

3. Add minced garlic, diced tomatoes, tomato paste, dried thyme, and dried oregano to the skillet. Stir to combine.

4. Season with salt and pepper to taste.

5. Reduce heat to low, cover, and simmer for 20-25 minutes, stirring occasionally, until vegetables are tender and flavors are blended.

6. Serve ratatouille warm, garnished with chopped fresh basil leaves and grated Parmesan cheese if desired.

7. Enjoy this classic French vegetable stew as a hearty and flavorful entree.

3. Spinach and Mushroom Quiche

Ingredients:

- ✓ 1 pie crust (store-bought or homemade)

GOUT DIET COOKBOOK

- ✓ 1 tablespoon olive oil

- ✓ 1 onion, diced

- ✓ 2 cups fresh spinach, chopped

- ✓ 1 cup mushrooms, sliced

- ✓ 4 eggs

- ✓ 1 cup milk or almond milk

- ✓ 1 cup shredded cheese (such as Swiss or Gruyère)

- ✓ Salt and pepper, to taste

- ✓ Fresh herbs (parsley, thyme), chopped (for garnish)

Instructions:

1. Preheat oven to 375°F (190°C).

2. In a skillet, heat olive oil over medium heat. Add diced onion and cook until translucent, about 3-4 minutes.

3. Add chopped spinach and sliced mushrooms to the skillet. Cook for 3-4 minutes until spinach is wilted and mushrooms are softened. Remove from heat.

4. In a bowl, whisk together eggs and milk until well combined. Season with salt and pepper.

5. Place pie crust in a pie dish. Spread spinach and mushroom mixture evenly over the bottom of the pie crust.

6. Sprinkle shredded cheese over the spinach and mushroom mixture.

7. Pour egg and milk mixture over the filling in the pie crust.

8. Bake in the preheated oven for 35-40 minutes or until quiche is set and golden brown on top.

9. Remove from oven and let cool slightly before slicing.

10. Garnish with chopped fresh herbs before serving.

11. Enjoy this savory and satisfying spinach and mushroom quiche as a delightful vegetable-forward dinner option.

Tips for Vegetable-Forward Entrees

- ✓ **Seasonal Produce:** Use fresh, seasonal vegetables for optimal flavor and nutrition.

- ✓ **Protein Boost:** Add protein-rich ingredients like beans, lentils, or tofu to vegetable-based dishes.

✓ **Diverse Flavors:** Experiment with herbs, spices, and sauces to enhance the taste of vegetable-forward entrees.

✓ **Meal Prep:** Prepare components of dishes ahead of time for quicker assembly on busy evenings.

✓ **Portion Control:** Enjoy these entrees with a side salad or whole grain bread to create a balanced meal.

These vegetable-forward entree recipes offer delicious and nutritious options for a satisfying dinner that supports a gout-friendly diet. Whether you prefer stuffed bell peppers with quinoa and black beans, ratatouille, or spinach and mushroom quiche, each recipe highlights the natural flavors and goodness of vegetables while providing wholesome meals that you'll love. Incorporate these dishes into your weekly dinner rotation for a well-rounded diet that promotes overall well-being and helps manage gout effectively.

6.3 Balanced Dinner Plates

Creating balanced dinner plates ensures you get a variety of nutrients while managing gout effectively. These recipes focus on incorporating lean proteins, wholesome grains, and plenty of vegetables to support your health goals and satisfy your taste buds. Here are some delicious and balanced dinner plate ideas to inspire your evening meals.

1. Grilled Chicken with Quinoa Pilaf and Steamed Broccoli

Ingredients:

- ✓ 4 boneless, skinless chicken breasts

- ✓ 1 cup quinoa, rinsed

- ✓ 2 cups vegetable broth or water

- ✓ 1 tablespoon olive oil

- ✓ 1 onion, diced

- ✓ 2 garlic cloves, minced

- ✓ 1/2 teaspoon ground cumin

- ✓ 1/2 teaspoon ground coriander

- ✓ Salt and pepper, to taste

- ✓ Fresh parsley or cilantro, chopped (for garnish)

- ✓ Fresh lemon wedges (for serving)

Instructions:

1. Preheat grill or grill pan over medium-high heat.

2. Season chicken breasts with salt, pepper, and a drizzle of olive oil. Grill chicken for 6-7 minutes per side, or until cooked through and no longer pink in the center.

3. In a saucepan, bring vegetable broth or water to a boil. Add rinsed quinoa, cover, and simmer for 15-20 minutes or until quinoa is cooked and liquid is absorbed.

4. Meanwhile, heat olive oil in a skillet over medium heat. Add diced onion and cook until translucent, about 3-4 minutes.

5. Add minced garlic, ground cumin, and ground coriander. Cook for another 1-2 minutes until fragrant.

6. Stir cooked quinoa into the skillet with onion and spices. Season with salt and pepper to taste.

7. Serve grilled chicken alongside quinoa pilaf and steamed broccoli.

8. Garnish with chopped fresh parsley or cilantro.

9. Squeeze fresh lemon juice over chicken and quinoa before serving.

10. Enjoy this balanced dinner plate with a mix of protein, whole grains, and vegetables.

2. Baked Cod with Roasted Vegetables and Brown Rice

Ingredients:

- ✓ 4 cod fillets

- ✓ 2 tablespoons olive oil

- ✓ 1 teaspoon paprika

- ✓ 1 teaspoon garlic powder

- ✓ 1 teaspoon dried thyme

- ✓ Salt and pepper, to taste

- ✓ 1 cup brown rice, rinsed

- ✓ 2 cups water or vegetable broth

- ✓ 1 sweet potato, diced

- ✓ 1 bunch asparagus, trimmed

- ✓ 1 tablespoon balsamic vinegar

- ✓ Fresh parsley, chopped (for garnish)

Instructions:

1. Preheat oven to 400°F (200°C).

2. Place cod fillets on a baking sheet lined with parchment paper. Drizzle with olive oil and sprinkle with paprika, garlic powder, dried thyme, salt, and pepper.

3. Bake cod in the preheated oven for 12-15 minutes, or until fish flakes easily with a fork.

4. In a saucepan, bring water or vegetable broth to a boil. Add rinsed brown rice, cover, and simmer for 40-45 minutes or until rice is tender and liquid is absorbed.

5. Toss diced sweet potato and trimmed asparagus with olive oil, salt, and pepper on a separate baking sheet.

6. Roast vegetables in the preheated oven for 20-25 minutes, stirring halfway through, until tender and lightly browned.

7. Drizzle roasted vegetables with balsamic vinegar and toss gently to coat.

8. Serve baked cod alongside brown rice and roasted vegetables.

9. Garnish with chopped fresh parsley.

10. Enjoy this nutritious and satisfying dinner plate with omega-3-rich fish, fiber-filled brown rice, and colorful vegetables.

3. Lentil and Vegetable Curry with Quinoa

Ingredients:

- ✓ 1 cup quinoa, rinsed
- ✓ 2 cups vegetable broth or water
- ✓ 1 tablespoon olive oil
- ✓ 1 onion, diced
- ✓ 2 garlic cloves, minced
- ✓ 1 tablespoon grated ginger
- ✓ 1 carrot, diced
- ✓ 1 bell pepper, diced
- ✓ 1 zucchini, diced

GOUT DIET COOKBOOK

- ✓ 1 can (15 ounces) lentils, drained and rinsed

- ✓ 1 can (14 ounces) diced tomatoes

- ✓ 1 can (14 ounces) coconut milk

- ✓ 2 teaspoons curry powder

- ✓ 1 teaspoon ground turmeric

- ✓ Salt and pepper, to taste

- ✓ Fresh cilantro, chopped (for garnish)

Instructions:

1. In a saucepan, bring vegetable broth or water to a boil. Add rinsed quinoa, cover, and simmer for 15-20 minutes or until quinoa is cooked and liquid is absorbed.

2. Meanwhile, heat olive oil in a large pot or Dutch oven over medium heat. Add diced onion and cook until translucent, about 3-4 minutes.

3. Add minced garlic and grated ginger. Cook for another 1-2 minutes until fragrant.

4. Stir in diced carrot, bell pepper, and zucchini. Cook for 5-7 minutes until vegetables begin to soften.

5. Add drained and rinsed lentils, diced tomatoes, coconut milk, curry powder, and ground turmeric to the pot. Stir to combine.

6. Season with salt and pepper to taste.

7. Bring curry to a boil, then reduce heat to low. Cover and simmer for 15-20 minutes, stirring occasionally, until vegetables are tender and flavors are blended.

8. Serve lentil and vegetable curry over cooked quinoa.

9. Garnish with chopped fresh cilantro.

10. Enjoy this plant-based and protein-rich dinner plate with a blend of hearty lentils, vibrant vegetables, and fluffy quinoa.

Tips for Balanced Dinner Plates

✓ **Protein Variety:** Incorporate lean proteins like chicken, fish, or plant-based options like lentils and beans.

✓ **Whole Grains:** Choose whole grains such as quinoa, brown rice, or whole wheat pasta for fiber and sustained energy.

- ✓ **Colorful Vegetables:** Aim for a variety of colorful vegetables to maximize nutrient intake and visual appeal.

- ✓ **Healthy Fats:** Include sources of healthy fats like olive oil, avocado, or nuts to support heart health.

- ✓ **Portion Control:** Balance your plate with appropriate portions of protein, grains, and vegetables for a well-rounded meal.

These balanced dinner plate recipes offer nutritious and satisfying options that support a gout-friendly diet. Whether you prefer grilled chicken with quinoa pilaf and steamed broccoli, baked cod with roasted vegetables and brown rice, or lentil and vegetable curry with quinoa, each recipe provides a mix of lean proteins, wholesome grains, and colorful vegetables for a well-rounded meal. Incorporate these dishes into your weekly dinner rotation to promote overall well-being and effectively manage gout while enjoying delicious and satisfying dinners.

CHAPTER SEVEN

SNACK AND APPETIZER RECIPES

7.1 Quick and Easy Snacks

Quick and easy snacks are perfect for satisfying cravings between meals or as a prelude to dinner. These recipes are not only delicious but also considerate of a gout-friendly diet, ensuring you can enjoy your snacks without worry. Here are some delightful ideas to tantalize your taste buds.

1. Avocado Toast with Cherry Tomatoes

Ingredients:

- ✓ 2 slices whole grain bread, toasted
- ✓ 1 ripe avocado
- ✓ 1 cup cherry tomatoes, halved
- ✓ Olive oil
- ✓ Lemon juice
- ✓ Salt and pepper, to taste
- ✓ Red pepper flakes (optional)
- ✓ Fresh basil leaves, chopped (for garnish)

Instructions:

1. Mash ripe avocado in a bowl until smooth. Season with a squeeze of lemon juice, salt, and pepper.

2. Spread mashed avocado evenly onto toasted whole grain bread slices.

3. Top with halved cherry tomatoes.

4. Drizzle with olive oil and sprinkle with red pepper flakes if desired.

5. Garnish with chopped fresh basil leaves.

6. Enjoy this simple yet satisfying avocado toast as a nutritious snack.

2. Greek Yogurt with Honey and Almonds

Ingredients:

- ✓ 1 cup Greek yogurt

- ✓ 1 tablespoon honey

- ✓ 2 tablespoons almonds, chopped

- ✓ Fresh berries (optional)

- ✓ Mint leaves, chopped (for garnish)

Instructions:

1. Spoon Greek yogurt into a serving bowl.

2. Drizzle honey over the yogurt.

3. Sprinkle chopped almonds on top.

4. Add fresh berries if desired.

5. Garnish with chopped mint leaves.

6. Enjoy this creamy and protein-rich Greek yogurt with honey and almonds for a sweet and crunchy snack.

3. Hummus with Veggie Sticks

Ingredients:

- ✓ 1 cup hummus (store-bought or homemade)

- ✓ Carrot sticks

- ✓ Cucumber slices

- ✓ Bell pepper strips (any color)

- ✓ Cherry tomatoes

Instructions:

1. Arrange carrot sticks, cucumber slices, bell pepper strips, and cherry tomatoes on a serving platter.

2. Serve with hummus for dipping.

3. Enjoy this refreshing and fiber-packed snack with a variety of colorful vegetables.

4. Trail Mix with Nuts and Dried Fruit

Ingredients:

- ✓ 1 cup mixed nuts (almonds, walnuts, cashews)

- ✓ 1/2 cup dried fruit (raisins, cranberries, apricots)

- ✓ 1/4 cup dark chocolate chips or chunks (optional)

Instructions:

1. Mix together mixed nuts, dried fruit, and dark chocolate chips or chunks in a bowl.

2. Portion into small snack bags or containers for easy grab-and-go snacks.

3. Enjoy this nutrient-dense trail mix as a satisfying and energy-boosting snack.

Tips for Quick and Easy Snacks

- ✓ **Portion Control:** Keep portions small to avoid overeating.

- ✓ **Nutrient Density:** Choose snacks that are rich in nutrients like fiber, protein, and healthy fats.

- ✓ **Hydration:** Pair snacks with a glass of water or herbal tea for hydration.

- ✓ **Preparation:** Prep snacks in advance for convenience during busy days.

- ✓ **Variety:** Explore different flavors and textures to keep snacks interesting and enjoyable.

These quick and easy snack recipes offer delicious options that align with a gout-friendly diet. Whether you prefer avocado toast with cherry tomatoes, Greek yogurt with honey and almonds, hummus with veggie sticks, or trail mix with nuts and dried fruit, each snack is designed to provide nourishment and satisfaction without compromising your health goals. Incorporate these snacks into your daily routine to keep cravings at bay and support overall well-being.

7.2 Healthy Appetizers

Here are some healthy appetizer recipes that are perfect for gatherings or as starters before a meal. These recipes are designed to be flavorful, satisfying, and mindful of a gout-friendly diet.

1. Caprese Skewers with Balsamic Glaze

Ingredients:

- Cherry tomatoes
- Fresh mozzarella balls
- Fresh basil leaves
- Balsamic glaze
- Salt and pepper, to taste
- Toothpicks or skewers

Instructions:

1. Thread a cherry tomato, a mozzarella ball, and a folded basil leaf onto each toothpick or skewer.

2. Arrange skewers on a serving platter.

3. Drizzle with balsamic glaze.

4. Season with salt and pepper to taste.

5. Serve these refreshing and elegant caprese skewers as a light and flavorful appetizer.

2. Cucumber Bites with Herbed Cream Cheese

Ingredients:

- ✓ 1 English cucumber, sliced into rounds
- ✓ 1/2 cup cream cheese, softened
- ✓ 1 tablespoon fresh dill, chopped
- ✓ 1 tablespoon fresh chives, chopped
- ✓ Salt and pepper, to taste
- ✓ Optional: Smoked salmon or prosciutto slices

Instructions:

1. In a bowl, mix together softened cream cheese, chopped fresh dill, chopped fresh chives, salt, and pepper until well combined.

2. Spread a dollop of herbed cream cheese onto each cucumber round.

3. Top with a small piece of smoked salmon or prosciutto if desired.

4. Arrange cucumber bites on a serving platter.

5. Enjoy these refreshing and creamy cucumber bites as a delightful appetizer option.

3. Stuffed Mini Bell Peppers with Herbed Goat Cheese

Ingredients:

- ✓ Mini bell peppers

- ✓ 4 ounces goat cheese, softened

- ✓ 1 tablespoon fresh parsley, chopped

- ✓ 1 tablespoon fresh basil, chopped

- ✓ 1 tablespoon fresh chives, chopped

- ✓ Salt and pepper, to taste

- ✓ Optional: Drizzle of balsamic glaze

Instructions:

1. Cut mini bell peppers in half lengthwise and remove seeds and membranes.

2. In a bowl, mix together softened goat cheese, chopped fresh parsley, chopped fresh basil, chopped fresh chives, salt, and pepper until smooth.

3. Spoon herbed goat cheese mixture into each mini bell pepper half.

4. Arrange stuffed mini bell peppers on a serving platter.

5. Drizzle with balsamic glaze if desired.

6. Serve these colorful and flavorful stuffed mini bell peppers as a tasty appetizer.

4. Smoked Salmon Cucumber Rolls

Ingredients:

- ✓ 1 English cucumber
- ✓ 4 ounces cream cheese, softened
- ✓ 4 ounces smoked salmon
- ✓ Fresh dill, for garnish
- ✓ Lemon zest (optional)

Instructions:

1. Using a vegetable peeler, slice the cucumber lengthwise into thin strips.

2. Spread a thin layer of softened cream cheese on each cucumber strip.

3. Place a slice of smoked salmon on top of the cream cheese.

4. Roll up the cucumber strip with the salmon inside.

5. Secure with a toothpick if necessary.

6. Garnish with fresh dill and lemon zest if desired.

7. Arrange smoked salmon cucumber rolls on a serving platter.

8. Enjoy these elegant and protein-rich appetizers with a burst of freshness.

Tips for Healthy Appetizers

- **Fresh Ingredients:** Use fresh herbs and high-quality ingredients for optimal flavor.

- **Presentation:** Arrange appetizers on a platter for an inviting presentation.

✓ **Customization:** Adjust recipes to accommodate dietary preferences and restrictions.

✓ **Balance:** Include a variety of textures and flavors to cater to different tastes.

✓ **Preparation:** Prepare appetizers ahead of time for convenience during gatherings.

These healthy appetizer recipes offer delicious options that align with a gout-friendly diet. Whether you prefer caprese skewers with balsamic glaze, cucumber bites with herbed cream cheese, stuffed mini bell peppers with herbed goat cheese, or smoked salmon cucumber rolls, each appetizer is designed to provide a delightful start to any meal or gathering. Incorporate these appetizers into your entertaining repertoire to impress guests and support your health goals with flavorful and satisfying choices.

7.3 Gout-Friendly Dips and Spreads

Creating gout-friendly dips and spreads allows you to enjoy flavorful accompaniments without compromising your health goals. These recipes are crafted to be delicious, satisfying, and mindful of ingredients that support managing gout. Here are some savory options to enhance your snacking or mealtime experience.

1. Guacamole with a Twist

Ingredients:

- ✓ 2 ripe avocados
- ✓ 1/2 cup Greek yogurt
- ✓ 1/4 cup red onion, finely chopped
- ✓ 1/4 cup cherry tomatoes, diced
- ✓ 1 jalapeño, seeded and finely chopped (optional)
- ✓ Juice of 1 lime
- ✓ Salt and pepper, to taste
- ✓ Fresh cilantro, chopped (for garnish)

Instructions:

1. In a bowl, mash ripe avocados until smooth.

2. Stir in Greek yogurt, finely chopped red onion, diced cherry tomatoes, and seeded and finely chopped jalapeño if using.

3. Squeeze lime juice over the mixture.

4. Season with salt and pepper to taste.

5. Garnish with chopped fresh cilantro.

6. Serve this creamy and flavorful guacamole with a twist with whole grain tortilla chips or vegetable sticks.

2. Baba Ganoush (Roasted Eggplant Dip)

Ingredients:

- ✓ 1 large eggplant
- ✓ 2 cloves garlic, minced
- ✓ Juice of 1 lemon
- ✓ 2 tablespoons tahini
- ✓ 2 tablespoons olive oil
- ✓ Salt and pepper, to taste
- ✓ Fresh parsley, chopped (for garnish)
- ✓ Optional: Smoked paprika or cumin for added flavor

GOUT DIET COOKBOOK

Instructions:

1. Preheat oven to 400°F (200°C).

2. Pierce eggplant with a fork in several places. Place eggplant on a baking sheet lined with parchment paper.

3. Roast eggplant in the preheated oven for 40-45 minutes or until tender and collapsed.

4. Remove eggplant from oven and let cool slightly. Peel off and discard skin.

5. In a food processor, combine roasted eggplant flesh, minced garlic, lemon juice, tahini, olive oil, salt, and pepper.

6. Blend until smooth and creamy.

7. Taste and adjust seasoning if needed. Add smoked paprika or cumin if desired for additional flavor.

8. Transfer baba ganoush to a serving bowl.

9. Drizzle with olive oil and garnish with chopped fresh parsley.

10. Serve this smoky and savory baba ganoush with pita bread or vegetable crudites.

3. Herbed White Bean Dip

Ingredients:

- ✓ 1 can (15 ounces) cannellini beans, drained and rinsed

- ✓ 2 tablespoons olive oil

- ✓ 1 tablespoon fresh lemon juice

- ✓ 1 garlic clove, minced

- ✓ 1 tablespoon fresh parsley, chopped

- ✓ 1 tablespoon fresh thyme leaves

- ✓ Salt and pepper, to taste

- ✓ Optional: Red pepper flakes for a hint of heat

Instructions:

1. In a food processor, combine cannellini beans, olive oil, fresh lemon juice, minced garlic, chopped fresh parsley, and fresh thyme leaves.

2. Blend until smooth and creamy.

3. Season with salt and pepper to taste.

4. For a hint of heat, add red pepper flakes if desired.

5. Transfer herbed white bean dip to a serving bowl.

6. Drizzle with olive oil and garnish with additional chopped fresh herbs.

7. Serve this creamy and herbaceous white bean dip with whole grain crackers or sliced vegetables.

Tips for Gout-Friendly Dips and Spreads

- ✓ **Bean Base:** Use beans like cannellini or chickpeas for fiber and protein.

- ✓ **Herbs and Citrus:** Incorporate fresh herbs and citrus juice for vibrant flavors.

- ✓ **Healthy Fats:** Choose olive oil or tahini for creamy texture and heart-healthy fats.

- ✓ **Customization:** Adjust recipes to suit your taste preferences and dietary needs.

- ✓ **Pairing:** Serve dips and spreads with whole grain options or vegetable sticks for added nutrition.

These gout-friendly dips and spreads offer flavorful options that complement your snacking or mealtime experience while supporting your health goals. Whether you prefer guacamole with a twist, baba ganoush (roasted eggplant dip), or herbed white bean dip, each recipe provides delicious and satisfying choices that align with managing gout effectively. Incorporate these dips and spreads into your repertoire to enjoy tasty and nutritious additions to your meals or gatherings.

CHAPTER EIGHT

DESSERT RECIPES

8.1 Low-Sugar Desserts

here are some delicious low-sugar dessert recipes that are mindful of managing gout and can satisfy your sweet tooth without overloading on sugar.

1. Berry Chia Seed Pudding

Ingredients:

- ✓ 1/4 cup chia seeds

- ✓ 1 cup unsweetened almond milk (or any milk of choice)

- ✓ 1 tablespoon honey or maple syrup (optional)

- ✓ 1/2 teaspoon vanilla extract

- ✓ Fresh berries (strawberries, blueberries, raspberries) for topping

Instructions:

1. In a bowl or jar, combine chia seeds, unsweetened almond milk, honey or maple syrup (if using), and vanilla extract.

2. Stir well to combine.

3. Cover and refrigerate for at least 2 hours or overnight until the mixture thickens and chia seeds absorb the liquid.

4. Stir well before serving.

5. Serve chia seed pudding topped with fresh berries.

6. Enjoy this creamy and satisfying dessert that's packed with fiber and omega-3 fatty acids.

2. Grilled Pineapple with Cinnamon and Honey

Ingredients:

- ✓ 1 pineapple, peeled, cored, and cut into rings

- ✓ 1 tablespoon honey

- ✓ 1/2 teaspoon ground cinnamon

- ✓ Fresh mint leaves, chopped (for garnish)

Instructions:

1. Preheat grill or grill pan over medium-high heat.

2. Grill pineapple rings for 2-3 minutes per side, or until grill marks appear and pineapple caramelizes slightly.

3. In a small bowl, mix together honey and ground cinnamon.

4. Brush grilled pineapple rings with honey-cinnamon mixture.

5. Serve grilled pineapple rings warm.

6. Garnish with chopped fresh mint leaves.

7. Enjoy this naturally sweet and caramelized dessert that's simple yet full of flavor.

3. Greek Yogurt Parfait with Fresh Berries

Ingredients:

- ✓ 1 cup Greek yogurt

- ✓ 1 tablespoon honey or maple syrup (optional)

- ✓ Fresh berries (strawberries, blueberries, raspberries)

- ✓ Granola or crushed nuts (optional)

GOUT DIET COOKBOOK

Instructions:

1. In a serving glass or bowl, layer Greek yogurt, honey or maple syrup (if using), fresh berries, and granola or crushed nuts (if using).

2. Repeat layers until the glass or bowl is filled.

3. Serve Greek yogurt parfait immediately.

4. Enjoy this creamy and protein-packed dessert that's rich in probiotics and antioxidants.

Tips for Low-Sugar Desserts

- ✓ **Natural Sweeteners:** Use honey, maple syrup, or ripe fruits to add sweetness.

- ✓ **Fruit Focus:** Incorporate fresh or frozen fruits for natural sweetness and fiber.

- ✓ **Portion Control:** Enjoy desserts in moderation to manage sugar intake.

- ✓ **Nutritional Balance:** Pair desserts with protein or healthy fats to stabilize blood sugar levels.

- ✓ **Creative Substitutions:** Experiment with alternative flours, like almond or coconut flour, for baking.

These low-sugar dessert recipes offer delicious options that align with managing gout and supporting overall health. Whether you prefer berry chia seed pudding, grilled pineapple with cinnamon and honey, or Greek yogurt parfait with fresh berries, each dessert provides a satisfying and nutritious way to indulge your sweet cravings without excessive sugar. Incorporate these desserts into your meal planning to enjoy guilt-free treats that contribute to your well-being and enjoyment of delicious flavors.

8.2 Fruit-Based Treats

Fruit-based treats offer a refreshing and naturally sweet way to satisfy cravings while staying mindful of managing gout. Here are some delightful recipes that highlight the natural flavors of fruits.

1. Mango Coconut Nice Cream

Ingredients:

- ✓ 2 ripe mangos, peeled and diced

- ✓ 1 can (14 ounces) full-fat coconut milk, chilled in the refrigerator overnight

- ✓ 2-3 tablespoons honey or maple syrup (optional)

- ✓ 1 teaspoon vanilla extract

- ✓ Fresh mango slices and shredded coconut for garnish

Instructions:

1. Place diced mango in a blender or food processor.

2. Scoop the thick coconut cream from the chilled coconut milk can (discard the liquid) and add it to the blender with the mango.

3. Add honey or maple syrup (if using) and vanilla extract.

4. Blend until smooth and creamy.

5. Transfer mango coconut mixture to a freezer-safe container.

6. Freeze for at least 4 hours or until firm, stirring occasionally.

7. Scoop mango coconut nice cream into bowls.

8. Garnish with fresh mango slices and shredded coconut.

9. Enjoy this creamy and tropical treat that's dairy-free and naturally sweetened.

2. Mixed Berry Sorbet

Ingredients:

- ✓ 3 cups mixed berries (strawberries, blueberries, raspberries)
- ✓ 1/4 cup honey or maple syrup
- ✓ Juice of 1 lemon
- ✓ Fresh mint leaves, chopped (for garnish)

Instructions:

1. In a blender or food processor, combine mixed berries, honey or maple syrup, and lemon juice.

2. Blend until smooth.

3. Pour berry mixture into a shallow dish or baking pan.

4. Cover with plastic wrap and freeze for 2-3 hours, or until edges are firm.

5. Remove from freezer and break up the frozen edges with a fork.

6. Return to freezer and freeze for another 2-3 hours, or until completely frozen.

7. Scoop mixed berry sorbet into bowls.

8. Garnish with chopped fresh mint leaves.

9. Enjoy this refreshing and antioxidant-rich sorbet that's perfect for hot days.

3. Grilled Peaches with Honey and Yogurt

Ingredients:

- ✓ 4 ripe peaches, halved and pitted

- ✓ Olive oil

- ✓ 2 tablespoons honey

- ✓ Greek yogurt for serving

- ✓ Fresh mint leaves, chopped (for garnish)

Instructions:

1. Preheat grill or grill pan over medium-high heat.

2. Brush peach halves lightly with olive oil.

3. Grill peaches for 3-4 minutes per side, or until grill marks appear and peaches are softened.

4. Drizzle grilled peach halves with honey.

5. Serve grilled peaches with a dollop of Greek yogurt.

6. Garnish with chopped fresh mint leaves.

7. Enjoy these warm and caramelized grilled peaches as a simple yet elegant dessert.

Tips for Fruit-Based Treats

✓ **Seasonal Varieties:** Use seasonal fruits for optimal flavor and freshness.

✓ **Frozen Options:** Substitute fresh fruits with frozen fruits for convenience.

✓ **Texture Play:** Experiment with different textures like smoothies, sorbets, or grilled fruits.

✓ **Nutritional Boost:** Add nuts or seeds for extra crunch and nutrients.

✓ **Family Fun:** Involve children in preparing and enjoying these fruity treats.

These fruit-based treat recipes offer delicious options that celebrate the natural sweetness of fruits while supporting your gout management goals. Whether you prefer mango coconut nice cream, mixed berry sorbet, or grilled peaches with honey and yogurt, each dessert provides a delightful and nutritious way to enjoy fruits in a variety of creative presentations. Incorporate these treats into your dessert repertoire to add color, flavor, and healthful benefits to your meals and special occasions.

8.3 Indulgent Yet Safe Sweets

Indulgent yet safe sweets provide a way to enjoy dessert without compromising health goals, especially for those managing gout. These recipes are crafted to be rich and satisfying while being mindful of ingredients that won't trigger gout flare-ups. Here are some delightful treats to savor.

1. Dark Chocolate Avocado Mousse

Ingredients:

- ✓ 2 ripe avocados

- ✓ 1/4 cup unsweetened cocoa powder

- ✓ 1/4 cup honey or maple syrup

- ✓ 1 teaspoon vanilla extract

- ✓ Pinch of salt

- ✓ Fresh berries for garnish

Instructions:

1. In a food processor or blender, combine avocados, unsweetened cocoa powder, honey or maple syrup, vanilla extract, and a pinch of salt.

2. Blend until smooth and creamy.

3. Taste and adjust sweetness if needed.

4. Spoon dark chocolate avocado mousse into serving bowls.

5. Chill in the refrigerator for at least 1 hour before serving.

6. Garnish with fresh berries.

7. Enjoy this rich and creamy mousse that's packed with healthy fats and antioxidants.

2. Baked Apple with Cinnamon and Walnuts

Ingredients:

GOUT DIET COOKBOOK

- ✓ 4 large apples, cored

- ✓ 1/4 cup walnuts, chopped

- ✓ 1 tablespoon honey

- ✓ 1 teaspoon ground cinnamon

- ✓ 1/4 teaspoon ground nutmeg

- ✓ Greek yogurt for serving (optional)

Instructions:

1. Preheat oven to 350°F (175°C).

2. Place cored apples in a baking dish.

3. In a small bowl, mix together chopped walnuts, honey, ground cinnamon, and ground nutmeg.

4. Stuff each apple with the walnut mixture.

5. Cover the baking dish with aluminum foil.

6. Bake for 25-30 minutes, or until apples are tender.

7. Remove from oven and let cool slightly.

8. Serve baked apples warm with a dollop of Greek yogurt if desired.

9. Enjoy this comforting and spiced dessert that's naturally sweetened and satisfying.

3. Almond Flour Brownies

Ingredients:

- ✓ 1 cup almond flour

- ✓ 1/4 cup unsweetened cocoa powder

- ✓ 1/2 teaspoon baking powder

- ✓ 1/4 teaspoon salt

- ✓ 2 large eggs

- ✓ 1/2 cup honey or maple syrup

- ✓ 1/4 cup coconut oil, melted

- ✓ 1 teaspoon vanilla extract

- ✓ 1/2 cup dark chocolate chips (optional)

Instructions:

1. Preheat oven to 350°F (175°C).

2. Line an 8x8-inch baking pan with parchment paper.

3. In a bowl, whisk together almond flour, unsweetened cocoa powder, baking powder, and salt.

4. In another bowl, beat eggs, honey or maple syrup, melted coconut oil, and vanilla extract until well combined.

5. Gradually add dry ingredients to wet ingredients, mixing until smooth.

6. Fold in dark chocolate chips if using.

7. Pour batter into the prepared baking pan.

8. Bake for 20-25 minutes, or until a toothpick inserted into the center comes out clean.

9. Let brownies cool in the pan before cutting into squares.

10. Enjoy these fudgy and indulgent brownies that are grain-free and lower in sugar.

Tips for Indulgent Yet Safe Sweets

✓ **Healthy Fats:** Use ingredients like avocados, nuts, and coconut oil for added nutrition.

- ✓ **Natural Sweeteners:** Opt for honey or maple syrup instead of refined sugars.

- ✓ **Portion Control:** Enjoy indulgent sweets in moderation to avoid overconsumption.

- ✓ **Nutrient Density:** Incorporate ingredients that add nutritional value, such as almond flour and dark chocolate.

- ✓ **Creative Garnishes:** Use fresh berries, nuts, or a dollop of yogurt to enhance flavor and presentation.

These indulgent yet safe sweets offer a way to enjoy rich and satisfying desserts while being mindful of managing gout. Whether you prefer dark chocolate avocado mousse, baked apples with cinnamon and walnuts, or almond flour brownies, each recipe provides a delicious and health-conscious option to satisfy your sweet tooth. Incorporate these treats into your dessert repertoire to enjoy decadent flavors and textures without compromising your health goals.

CHAPTER NINE

SPECIAL DIET CONSIDERATIONS

9.1 Vegetarian and Vegan Options

Here's a detailed exploration of vegetarian and vegan options, considering special diet considerations for those managing gout or simply looking to incorporate more plant-based meals into their diet.

Special Diet Considerations

9.1 Vegetarian and Vegan Options

Choosing vegetarian or vegan options can be a rewarding journey towards better health and sustainability. Whether you're exploring these dietary choices for ethical reasons, health benefits, or managing conditions like gout, there are plenty of delicious and nutritious options to explore.

Why Choose Vegetarian or Vegan?

Vegetarian diets exclude meat, poultry, and seafood, while vegan diets exclude all animal products, including dairy and eggs. These diets are rich in fruits, vegetables, legumes, nuts, seeds, and whole grains, providing essential nutrients like fiber, vitamins, minerals, and antioxidants. Studies suggest that vegetarian and vegan diets may offer various health benefits, including lower risk of heart disease, hypertension, type 2 diabetes, and certain cancers.

Vegetarian and Vegan Protein Sources

Protein is essential for overall health and well-being, and it can be easily obtained from plant-based sources. Here are some excellent sources of protein for vegetarians and vegans:

- ✓ **Legumes:** Lentils, chickpeas, black beans, and peas are rich in protein, fiber, and various vitamins and minerals.

- ✓ **Tofu and Tempeh:** Soy-based products like tofu and tempeh are versatile and protein-rich.

- ✓ **Quinoa:** This ancient grain is a complete protein, containing all nine essential amino acids.

- ✓ **Nuts and Seeds:** Almonds, walnuts, chia seeds, and hemp seeds are packed with protein, healthy fats, and micronutrients.

Essential Nutrients to Consider

When following a vegetarian or vegan diet, it's important to ensure adequate intake of certain nutrients that may be more challenging to obtain from plant-based sources:

- ✓ **Vitamin B12:** Found in fortified foods or supplements, vitamin B12 is crucial for nerve function and red blood cell production.

- ✓ **Iron:** Plant-based iron sources include lentils, beans, spinach, and fortified cereals. Pairing these foods with vitamin C-rich foods enhances iron absorption.

- ✓ **Omega-3 Fatty Acids:** Flaxseeds, chia seeds, and walnuts are good sources of plant-based omega-3 fatty acids, important for heart health and inflammation management.

Vegetarian and Vegan Recipes

Here are some delicious and nutritious vegetarian and vegan recipes that are suitable for those managing gout or looking to explore plant-based options:

1. Chickpea and Spinach Curry (Vegetarian)

Ingredients:

- ✓ 1 tablespoon olive oil

- ✓ 1 onion, chopped

- ✓ 3 garlic cloves, minced

- ✓ 1 tablespoon ginger, minced

- ✓ 1 teaspoon ground cumin

- ✓ 1 teaspoon ground coriander

- ✓ 1/2 teaspoon turmeric

- ✓ 1/4 teaspoon cayenne pepper (optional)

- ✓ 1 can (15 ounces) chickpeas, drained and rinsed

- ✓ 1 can (14 ounces) diced tomatoes

- ✓ 1 can (14 ounces) coconut milk

- ✓ 3 cups fresh spinach

- ✓ Salt and pepper, to taste

- ✓ Fresh cilantro, chopped (for garnish)

- ✓ Cooked rice or naan bread, for serving

Instructions:

1. Heat olive oil in a large skillet over medium heat.

2. Add chopped onion and sauté until softened, about 5 minutes.

3. Add minced garlic and ginger, and sauté for another minute until fragrant.

4. Stir in ground cumin, ground coriander, turmeric, and cayenne pepper (if using), and cook for 1 minute.

5. Add drained and rinsed chickpeas, diced tomatoes (with juices), and coconut milk to the skillet.

6. Bring to a simmer and cook for 10-15 minutes, stirring occasionally, until the sauce thickens slightly.

7. Add fresh spinach and cook until wilted.

8. Season with salt and pepper to taste.

9. Garnish with chopped fresh cilantro.

10. Serve chickpea and spinach curry over cooked rice or with naan bread.

2. Lentil Walnut Tacos (Vegan)

Ingredients:

- ✓ 1 cup green or brown lentils, rinsed

- ✓ 2 cups vegetable broth or water

- ✓ 1 tablespoon olive oil

- ✓ 1 onion, chopped

- ✓ 2 garlic cloves, minced

- ✓ 1 tablespoon chili powder

- ✓ 1 teaspoon ground cumin

- ✓ 1/2 teaspoon paprika

- ✓ 1/4 teaspoon cayenne pepper (optional)

- ✓ Salt and pepper, to taste

- ✓ 1/2 cup walnuts, chopped

- ✓ Corn or flour tortillas

- ✓ Toppings: Shredded lettuce, diced tomatoes, avocado slices, salsa, lime wedges

Instructions:

1. In a medium saucepan, combine lentils and vegetable broth or water.

2. Bring to a boil, then reduce heat to low, cover, and simmer for 20-25 minutes, or until lentils are tender and liquid is absorbed.

3. Heat olive oil in a large skillet over medium heat.

4. Add chopped onion and sauté until softened, about 5 minutes.

5. Add minced garlic, chili powder, ground cumin, paprika, cayenne pepper (if using), salt, and pepper, and cook for 1 minute until fragrant.

6. Stir in chopped walnuts and cooked lentils, and cook for 5-7 minutes, stirring occasionally, until heated through and flavors are combined.

7. Warm tortillas in a dry skillet or microwave.

8. Spoon lentil walnut mixture onto tortillas.

9. Top with shredded lettuce, diced tomatoes, avocado slices, salsa, and a squeeze of lime juice.

10. Serve lentil walnut tacos with your favorite toppings.

Tips for Vegetarian and Vegan Options

✓ **Balanced Meals:** Include a variety of colorful vegetables, whole grains, and protein-rich legumes or tofu.

✓ **Plant-Based Protein:** Experiment with different sources of plant-based protein to ensure a well-rounded diet.

- ✓ **Cooking Techniques:** Explore cooking methods like roasting, sautéing, and grilling to enhance flavors and textures.

- ✓ **Meal Planning:** Plan meals ahead to ensure nutritional balance and variety throughout the week.

- ✓ **Recipe Adaptations:** Modify recipes based on personal taste preferences and ingredient availability.

Vegetarian and vegan diets offer a wide range of delicious and nutritious options that can support your health goals, including managing conditions like gout. By incorporating diverse plant-based foods rich in vitamins, minerals, and antioxidants, you can enjoy flavorful meals while promoting overall well-being. Whether you're preparing chickpea and spinach curry, lentil walnut tacos, or exploring other vegetarian and vegan recipes, each dish provides a satisfying and health-conscious choice for your dietary journey. Embrace the abundance of plant-based ingredients to create meals that nourish both body and soul.

9.2 Gluten-Free Recipes

Here's an extensive section on gluten-free recipes, tailored for those who need to manage gout and other health considerations.

Special Diet Considerations

A gluten-free diet is essential for individuals with celiac disease or gluten sensitivity. It's also beneficial for those looking to reduce inflammation, which can be crucial for managing gout. Gluten-free recipes can be delicious, nutritious, and easy to prepare. Here, we'll explore some delightful gluten-free recipes that are gout-friendly and packed with flavor.

Understanding Gluten-Free Ingredients

When adopting a gluten-free diet, it's important to be aware of hidden sources of gluten. Gluten is found in wheat, barley, rye, and their derivatives. Here are some common gluten-free grains and flours:

- ✓ **Quinoa:** A complete protein that's versatile and nutrient-dense.

- ✓ **Rice:** Both white and brown rice are gluten-free staples.

- ✓ **Buckwheat:** Despite its name, buckwheat is gluten-free and perfect for pancakes and porridge.

- ✓ **Cornmeal:** Great for polenta and gluten-free baking.

- ✓ **Almond Flour:** Adds moisture and a nutty flavor to baked goods.

- ✓ **Coconut Flour:** A high-fiber flour that works well in many recipes.

1. Gluten-Free Breakfast Recipes

Quinoa Breakfast Bowl

Ingredients:

- ✓ 1 cup quinoa, rinsed

- ✓ 2 cups water or milk of choice

- ✓ 1 tablespoon honey or maple syrup

- ✓ 1 teaspoon vanilla extract

- ✓ Fresh berries (strawberries, blueberries, raspberries)

- ✓ Nuts and seeds (almonds, chia seeds, flaxseeds)

- ✓ Coconut flakes (optional)

Instructions:

1. In a medium saucepan, combine quinoa and water or milk.

2. Bring to a boil, then reduce heat to low, cover, and simmer for 15 minutes or until quinoa is tender and liquid is absorbed.

3. Stir in honey or maple syrup and vanilla extract.

4. Spoon quinoa into bowls and top with fresh berries, nuts, seeds, and coconut flakes.

5. Enjoy this protein-packed and flavorful breakfast that keeps you full and energized.

2. Sweet Potato Hash with Avocado

Ingredients:

- ✓ 2 large sweet potatoes, peeled and diced

- ✓ 1 tablespoon olive oil

- ✓ 1 onion, chopped

GOUT DIET COOKBOOK

- ✓ 1 red bell pepper, chopped
- ✓ 2 garlic cloves, minced
- ✓ 1 teaspoon ground cumin
- ✓ 1/2 teaspoon smoked paprika
- ✓ Salt and pepper, to taste
- ✓ 1 avocado, sliced
- ✓ Fresh cilantro, chopped (for garnish)

Instructions:

1. Heat olive oil in a large skillet over medium heat.

2. Add diced sweet potatoes and cook for 10-12 minutes, stirring occasionally, until tender and lightly browned.

3. Add chopped onion, red bell pepper, and minced garlic, and sauté for 5-7 minutes until vegetables are softened.

4. Stir in ground cumin, smoked paprika, salt, and pepper.

5. Cook for another 2-3 minutes until spices are well combined.

6. Serve sweet potato hash topped with avocado slices and chopped fresh cilantro.

7. Enjoy this hearty and nutritious breakfast that's rich in vitamins and healthy fats.

3. Gluten-Free Lunch Recipes

Quinoa and Black Bean Salad

Ingredients:

- ✓ 1 cup quinoa, rinsed

- ✓ 2 cups water

- ✓ 1 can (15 ounces) black beans, drained and rinsed

- ✓ 1 cup cherry tomatoes, halved

- ✓ 1 red bell pepper, chopped

- ✓ 1/4 cup red onion, finely chopped

- ✓ 1/4 cup fresh cilantro, chopped

- ✓ 1/4 cup olive oil

- ✓ Juice of 2 limes

✓ Salt and pepper, to taste

Instructions:

1. In a medium saucepan, combine quinoa and water.

2. Bring to a boil, then reduce heat to low, cover, and simmer for 15 minutes or until quinoa is tender and liquid is absorbed.

3. In a large bowl, combine cooked quinoa, black beans, cherry tomatoes, red bell pepper, red onion, and fresh cilantro.

4. In a small bowl, whisk together olive oil, lime juice, salt, and pepper.

5. Pour dressing over the quinoa salad and toss to combine.

6. Serve chilled or at room temperature.

7. Enjoy this refreshing and protein-rich salad that's perfect for a light lunch.

4. Zucchini Noodles with Pesto

Ingredients:

✓ 4 medium zucchinis, spiralized into noodles

- ✓ 1/2 cup fresh basil leaves

- ✓ 1/4 cup pine nuts or walnuts

- ✓ 2 garlic cloves

- ✓ 1/4 cup olive oil

- ✓ 1/4 cup nutritional yeast (for a cheesy flavor)

- ✓ Salt and pepper, to taste

- ✓ Cherry tomatoes, halved (for garnish)

Instructions:

1. In a food processor, combine fresh basil leaves, pine nuts or walnuts, garlic cloves, olive oil, nutritional yeast, salt, and pepper.

2. Process until smooth, adding more olive oil if needed to reach desired consistency.

3. In a large bowl, toss zucchini noodles with the pesto until well coated.

4. Garnish with halved cherry tomatoes.

5. Serve immediately and enjoy this light, fresh, and gluten-free lunch that's bursting with flavor.

5. Gluten-Free Dinner Recipes

Baked Lemon Herb Chicken with Roasted Vegetables

Ingredients:

- ✓ 4 boneless, skinless chicken breasts

- ✓ 2 tablespoons olive oil

- ✓ Juice of 2 lemons

- ✓ 2 garlic cloves, minced

- ✓ 1 teaspoon dried oregano

- ✓ 1 teaspoon dried thyme

- ✓ Salt and pepper, to taste

- ✓ 2 cups mixed vegetables (carrots, broccoli, bell peppers), chopped

Instructions:

1. Preheat oven to 375°F (190°C).

2. In a small bowl, whisk together olive oil, lemon juice, minced garlic, dried oregano, dried thyme, salt, and pepper.

3. Place chicken breasts in a baking dish and pour the lemon herb mixture over them, turning to coat evenly.

4. Arrange mixed vegetables around the chicken in the baking dish.

5. Bake for 25-30 minutes, or until chicken is cooked through and vegetables are tender.

6. Serve baked lemon herb chicken with roasted vegetables.

7. Enjoy this flavorful and easy gluten-free dinner that's perfect for busy weeknights.

6. Cauliflower Rice Stir-Fry

Ingredients:

- ✓ 1 head of cauliflower, grated or processed into rice-sized pieces

- ✓ 2 tablespoons olive oil

- ✓ 1 onion, chopped

- ✓ 2 garlic cloves, minced

GOUT DIET COOKBOOK

- ✓ 1 cup mixed vegetables (carrots, peas, bell peppers), chopped

- ✓ 2 tablespoons gluten-free soy sauce or tamari

- ✓ 1 tablespoon sesame oil

- ✓ 2 green onions, chopped (for garnish)

- ✓ Sesame seeds (for garnish)

Instructions:

1. Heat olive oil in a large skillet or wok over medium heat.

2. Add chopped onion and minced garlic, and sauté for 2-3 minutes until fragrant.

3. Add mixed vegetables and cook for 5-7 minutes until tender.

4. Stir in grated cauliflower and cook for another 5-7 minutes, stirring occasionally, until cauliflower is tender.

5. Add gluten-free soy sauce or tamari and sesame oil, and stir to combine.

6. Cook for another 2-3 minutes until flavors are well combined.

7. Garnish with chopped green onions and sesame seeds.

8. Serve hot and enjoy this nutritious and satisfying gluten-free stir-fry.

Tips for Gluten-Free Cooking

- ✓ **Read Labels:** Always check food labels for hidden sources of gluten.

- ✓ **Cross-Contamination:** Avoid cross-contamination by using separate utensils and cookware for gluten-free foods.

- ✓ **Experiment with Flours:** Use a variety of gluten-free flours like almond, coconut, and rice flour for different textures and flavors in baking.

- ✓ **Whole Foods:** Focus on whole, unprocessed foods to naturally avoid gluten.

✓ **Flavor Enhancers:** Use fresh herbs, spices, and citrus juices to enhance the flavor of gluten-free dishes.

Adopting a gluten-free diet doesn't mean sacrificing flavor or variety. With these gluten-free recipes, you can enjoy delicious and nutritious meals that support your health and help manage conditions like gout. From quinoa breakfast bowls and sweet potato hash to quinoa salads, zucchini noodles with pesto, baked lemon herb chicken, and cauliflower rice stir-fry, each dish is crafted to be satisfying and mindful of your dietary needs. Embrace the world of gluten-free cooking and discover how flavorful and diverse your meals can be.

9.3 Dairy-Free Alternatives

Whether you're lactose intolerant, allergic to dairy, or simply choosing to exclude dairy from your diet, dairy-free alternatives can be both delicious and nutritious. In this section, we'll explore a variety of dairy-free substitutes and recipes that cater to those managing gout or anyone looking to reduce their dairy intake.

Benefits of Going Dairy-Free

Eliminating dairy from your diet can have several benefits, including:

- ✓ **Reduced Inflammation:** For some people, dairy can cause inflammation, which can exacerbate conditions like gout.

- ✓ **Improved Digestion:** Many individuals find that removing dairy improves their digestive health, reducing symptoms like bloating and gas.

- ✓ **Clearer Skin:** Some people experience clearer skin and fewer acne breakouts after going dairy-free.

Dairy-Free Substitutes

Here are some popular dairy-free substitutes to use in cooking and baking:

- ✓ **Milk Alternatives:** Almond milk, soy milk, oat milk, coconut milk, and rice milk are all excellent substitutes for cow's milk. They can be used in everything from cereal to baking.

- ✓ **Butter Alternatives:** Coconut oil, olive oil, and plant-based butters made from nuts or seeds can replace butter in most recipes.

✓ **Cheese Alternatives:** Nutritional yeast adds a cheesy flavor to dishes. Plant-based cheeses made from nuts (like cashew cheese) are also widely available.

✓ **Yogurt Alternatives:** Almond, soy, and coconut-based yogurts provide a creamy texture and can be used in parfaits, smoothies, and as a base for dressings.

Dairy-Free Breakfast Recipes

1. Almond Milk Chia Pudding

Ingredients:

✓ 1 cup almond milk

✓ 3 tablespoons chia seeds

✓ 1 tablespoon maple syrup or honey

✓ 1/2 teaspoon vanilla extract

✓ Fresh berries and nuts for topping

Instructions:

1. In a bowl, whisk together almond milk, chia seeds, maple syrup or honey, and vanilla extract.

2. Cover and refrigerate for at least 4 hours or overnight, stirring occasionally to prevent clumping.

3. Once the chia seeds have absorbed the liquid and the mixture has thickened, give it a good stir.

4. Serve topped with fresh berries and nuts for a nutritious and filling breakfast.

2. Coconut Milk Smoothie Bowl

Ingredients:

- ✓ 1 cup coconut milk

- ✓ 1 frozen banana

- ✓ 1/2 cup frozen berries

- ✓ 1 tablespoon almond butter

- ✓ 1 teaspoon chia seeds

✓ Fresh fruit, granola, and coconut flakes for topping

Instructions:

1. In a blender, combine coconut milk, frozen banana, frozen berries, almond butter, and chia seeds.

2. Blend until smooth and creamy.

3. Pour into a bowl and top with fresh fruit, granola, and coconut flakes.

4. Enjoy this creamy and refreshing smoothie bowl that's perfect for a dairy-free breakfast.

Dairy-Free Lunch Recipes

1. Creamy Avocado Pasta

Ingredients:

✓ 12 ounces gluten-free pasta

✓ 2 ripe avocados

✓ 1/4 cup olive oil

✓ 2 cloves garlic

- ✓ Juice of 1 lemon

- ✓ Salt and pepper, to taste

- ✓ Cherry tomatoes, halved

- ✓ Fresh basil, chopped

Instructions:

1. Cook the gluten-free pasta according to package instructions.

2. While the pasta is cooking, combine avocados, olive oil, garlic, lemon juice, salt, and pepper in a food processor. Blend until smooth and creamy.

3. Drain the pasta and return it to the pot.

4. Add the avocado sauce to the pasta and toss to coat.

5. Stir in halved cherry tomatoes and chopped fresh basil.

6. Serve immediately and enjoy this rich and creamy pasta dish without any dairy.

2. Dairy-Free Chickpea Salad

Ingredients:

- ✓ 1 can (15 ounces) chickpeas, drained and rinsed

- ✓ 1/4 cup red onion, finely chopped

- ✓ 1 celery stalk, chopped

- ✓ 1/4 cup vegan mayonnaise

- ✓ 1 tablespoon lemon juice

- ✓ 1 teaspoon Dijon mustard

- ✓ Salt and pepper, to taste

- ✓ Fresh parsley, chopped (for garnish)

- ✓ Lettuce leaves or gluten-free bread, for serving

Instructions:

1. In a bowl, mash the chickpeas with a fork until partially smashed but still chunky.

2. Add chopped red onion, celery, vegan mayonnaise, lemon juice, Dijon mustard, salt, and pepper.

3. Mix well to combine.

4. Serve the chickpea salad on lettuce leaves or gluten-free bread.

5. Garnish with chopped fresh parsley.

6. Enjoy this protein-packed and satisfying lunch that's dairy-free and delicious.

Dairy-Free Dinner Recipes

1. Coconut Curry with Vegetables

Ingredients:

- ✓ 1 tablespoon coconut oil

- ✓ 1 onion, chopped

- ✓ 2 garlic cloves, minced

- ✓ 1 tablespoon ginger, minced

- ✓ 1 tablespoon curry powder

- ✓ 1 can (14 ounces) coconut milk

- ✓ 2 cups mixed vegetables (carrots, bell peppers, broccoli), chopped

- ✓ 1 can (15 ounces) chickpeas, drained and rinsed

- ✓ Salt and pepper, to taste

- ✓ Fresh cilantro, chopped (for garnish)

✓ Cooked rice or quinoa, for serving

Instructions:

1. Heat coconut oil in a large skillet over medium heat.

2. Add chopped onion and sauté until softened, about 5 minutes.

3. Add minced garlic and ginger, and cook for another minute until fragrant.

4. Stir in curry powder and cook for 1 minute.

5. Pour in coconut milk and bring to a simmer.

6. Add mixed vegetables and chickpeas, and cook for 10-15 minutes until vegetables are tender.

7. Season with salt and pepper to taste.

8. Serve the coconut curry over cooked rice or quinoa.

9. Garnish with chopped fresh cilantro.

10. Enjoy this flavorful and creamy curry that's completely dairy-free.

2. Dairy-Free Stuffed Bell Peppers

Ingredients:

GOUT DIET COOKBOOK

- ✓ 4 bell peppers, tops cut off and seeds removed

- ✓ 1 tablespoon olive oil

- ✓ 1 onion, chopped

- ✓ 2 garlic cloves, minced

- ✓ 1 cup cooked quinoa

- ✓ 1 can (15 ounces) black beans, drained and rinsed

- ✓ 1 cup corn kernels

- ✓ 1 teaspoon cumin

- ✓ 1 teaspoon chili powder

- ✓ Salt and pepper, to taste

- ✓ 1/2 cup tomato sauce

- ✓ Fresh cilantro, chopped (for garnish)

Instructions:

1. Preheat oven to 375°F (190°C).

2. In a large skillet, heat olive oil over medium heat.

3. Add chopped onion and sauté until softened, about 5 minutes.

4. Add minced garlic and cook for another minute until fragrant.

5. Stir in cooked quinoa, black beans, corn kernels, cumin, chili powder, salt, and pepper.

6. Add tomato sauce and mix well to combine.

7. Stuff the bell peppers with the quinoa mixture and place them in a baking dish.

8. Cover with aluminum foil and bake for 25-30 minutes until the peppers are tender.

9. Remove from oven and let cool slightly.

10. Garnish with chopped fresh cilantro.

11. Serve and enjoy these hearty and nutritious stuffed bell peppers that are dairy-free.

Tips for Dairy-Free Cooking

✓ **Experiment with Flavors:** Use herbs, spices, and citrus to enhance the flavor of your dairy-free dishes.

✓ **Texture Matters:** Find dairy-free substitutes that mimic the texture of dairy products, such as creamy coconut milk or rich avocado.

✓ **Check Labels:** Be vigilant about checking food labels for hidden dairy ingredients.

✓ **Homemade Alternatives:** Make your own dairy-free alternatives like nut milk or cashew cheese to control ingredients and ensure freshness.

✓ **Nutritional Balance:** Ensure you're getting enough calcium and vitamin D from other sources like leafy greens, fortified plant-based milks, and supplements if necessary.

Adopting a dairy-free diet can open up a world of flavorful and nutritious possibilities. These dairy-free recipes are designed to be both satisfying and supportive of your health, particularly for those managing gout. From almond milk chia pudding and coconut milk smoothie bowls for breakfast, to creamy avocado pasta and chickpea salad for lunch, and coconut curry with vegetables and stuffed bell peppers for dinner, you can enjoy a variety of delicious meals without dairy. Embrace the creativity and flavors of dairy-free cooking and discover how enjoyable and fulfilling this lifestyle can be.

CHAPTER TEN

BEVERAGES

10.1 Hydrating Drinks

Staying hydrated is crucial for overall health and particularly important for managing gout. Proper hydration helps to flush uric acid from the body, potentially reducing the frequency and severity of gout attacks. In this section, we'll explore a variety of delicious and hydrating drinks that not only quench your thirst but also support your health.

The Importance of Hydration

Hydration plays a vital role in maintaining bodily functions, including:

- ✓ **Regulating Body Temperature:** Water helps to regulate your body temperature, especially during exercise or hot weather.

- ✓ **Lubricating Joints:** Adequate hydration keeps your joints well-lubricated, which is particularly beneficial for individuals with gout.

- ✓ **Supporting Kidney Function:** Drinking enough fluids helps your kidneys filter waste products, including excess uric acid.

- ✓ **Aiding Digestion:** Water is essential for digestion and helps prevent constipation.

Simple and Refreshing Hydrating Drinks

1. Lemon Water

Lemon water is a simple yet incredibly refreshing drink. It's an excellent way to start your day or enjoy as a pick-me-up throughout the day.

Ingredients:

- ✓ 1 lemon

- ✓ 1 liter of water

- ✓ Ice cubes (optional)

- ✓ Fresh mint leaves (optional)

Instructions:

1. Slice the lemon into thin rounds.

2. Add the lemon slices to a pitcher of water.

3. For an extra burst of flavor, add a few fresh mint leaves.

4. Refrigerate for at least 30 minutes to allow the flavors to infuse.

5. Serve over ice if desired.

6. Enjoy this invigorating and hydrating drink.

2. Cucumber Mint Water

Cucumber mint water is not only hydrating but also incredibly cooling, making it perfect for hot days or post-workout refreshment.

Ingredients:

- ✓ 1 cucumber
- ✓ A handful of fresh mint leaves
- ✓ 1 liter of water
- ✓ Ice cubes (optional)

Instructions:

1. Slice the cucumber into thin rounds.

2. Add the cucumber slices and mint leaves to a pitcher of water.

3. Refrigerate for at least 30 minutes to allow the flavors to infuse.

4. Serve over ice if desired.

5. Enjoy this refreshing and hydrating beverage that's great for detoxing and cooling down.

3. Herbal Infusions

Herbal infusions, also known as herbal teas, are a wonderful way to stay hydrated and benefit from the natural properties of herbs. Here are a few herbal infusions that are particularly good for hydration and gout management:

Peppermint Tea:

- ✓ **Ingredients:** Fresh or dried peppermint leaves, hot water.

- ✓ **Instructions:** Steep a handful of fresh peppermint leaves or a teaspoon of dried peppermint in hot water for 5-10 minutes. Strain and enjoy hot or iced.

Chamomile Tea:

- ✓ **Ingredients:** Dried chamomile flowers, hot water.

- ✓ **Instructions:** Steep a tablespoon of dried chamomile flowers in hot water for 5-10 minutes. Strain and enjoy hot or iced.

Ginger Tea:

- ✓ **Ingredients:** Fresh ginger root, hot water, lemon, and honey (optional).

- ✓ **Instructions:** Slice a piece of fresh ginger root and steep in hot water for 10 minutes. Add a squeeze of lemon and a teaspoon of honey if desired. Enjoy hot or iced.

Hydrating Smoothies

Smoothies are a fantastic way to hydrate while also getting a boost of nutrients. Here are a few hydrating smoothie recipes:

1. Tropical Hydration Smoothie

Ingredients:

- ✓ 1 cup coconut water

- ✓ 1 cup frozen pineapple chunks

- ✓ 1 banana

- ✓ 1/2 cup Greek yogurt or a dairy-free alternative

- ✓ 1 tablespoon chia seeds

- ✓ Ice cubes (optional)

Instructions:

1. Combine all ingredients in a blender.

2. Blend until smooth.

3. Add ice cubes if you prefer a thicker, colder smoothie.

4. Enjoy this tropical, hydrating smoothie packed with electrolytes and vitamins.

2. Berry Coconut Water Smoothie

Ingredients:

- ✓ 1 cup coconut water

- ✓ 1 cup mixed berries (strawberries, blueberries, raspberries)

- ✓ 1/2 cup Greek yogurt or a dairy-free alternative

- ✓ 1 tablespoon flaxseeds

- ✓ Ice cubes (optional)

Instructions:

1. Combine all ingredients in a blender.

2. Blend until smooth.

3. Add ice cubes if you prefer a thicker, colder smoothie.

4. Enjoy this antioxidant-rich and hydrating smoothie.

Infused Waters

Infused waters are a delightful way to add flavor to your hydration routine without any added sugars or artificial ingredients. Here are some combinations to try:

Citrus Bliss:

- ✓ **Ingredients:** Slices of orange, lemon, and lime.

- ✓ **Instructions:** Add the citrus slices to a pitcher of water and let it infuse for at least 30 minutes before serving.

Berry Delight:

- ✓ **Ingredients:** Fresh strawberries, blueberries, and raspberries.

- ✓ **Instructions:** Add the berries to a pitcher of water and let it infuse for at least 30 minutes before serving.

Tropical Twist:

- ✓ **Ingredients:** Slices of pineapple and mango.

- ✓ **Instructions:** Add the fruit slices to a pitcher of water and let it infuse for at least 30 minutes before serving.

Staying hydrated is key to managing gout and maintaining overall health. With these hydrating drink recipes, you can enjoy a variety of flavors while keeping your body well-hydrated. From simple lemon water and cucumber mint water to herbal infusions and nutrient-packed smoothies, these beverages are designed to quench your thirst and support your wellness. Embrace these delicious hydrating drinks as part of your daily routine and feel the benefits of staying properly hydrated.

10.2 Anti-Inflammatory Teas and Tonics

For individuals managing gout, reducing inflammation is crucial. Incorporating anti-inflammatory teas and tonics into your diet can provide soothing relief and contribute to overall wellness. This section explores a variety of beverages that are not only delicious but also packed with ingredients known for their anti-inflammatory properties.

The Power of Anti-Inflammatory Ingredients

Certain ingredients are renowned for their ability to combat inflammation and support joint health. Key players include:

- ✓ **Turmeric:** Contains curcumin, a potent anti-inflammatory compound.

- ✓ **Ginger:** Known for its ability to reduce inflammation and improve digestion.

- ✓ **Green Tea:** Rich in antioxidants and polyphenols that help reduce inflammation.

- ✓ **Cinnamon:** Has anti-inflammatory and antioxidant properties.

- ✓ **Chamomile:** Offers soothing effects and helps reduce inflammation.

- ✓ **Peppermint:** Provides a cooling sensation and has anti-inflammatory benefits.

Anti-Inflammatory Teas

1. Turmeric and Ginger Tea

This golden tea is a powerhouse of anti-inflammatory benefits, combining turmeric and ginger for a soothing, healing drink.

Ingredients:

- ✓ 1 teaspoon turmeric powder or grated fresh turmeric

- ✓ 1 teaspoon grated fresh ginger

- ✓ 2 cups water

- ✓ 1 tablespoon honey (optional)

- ✓ Juice of half a lemon (optional)

✓ A pinch of black pepper (enhances curcumin absorption)

Instructions:

1. Bring water to a boil in a small pot.

2. Add turmeric and ginger, reduce heat, and let simmer for 10 minutes.

3. Strain the tea into a cup.

4. Add honey and lemon juice if desired.

5. Stir in a pinch of black pepper to enhance the absorption of curcumin.

6. Enjoy this warming, anti-inflammatory tea.

2. Green Tea with Lemon and Honey

Green tea is rich in antioxidants, and adding lemon and honey boosts its anti-inflammatory properties and makes it even more delicious.

Ingredients:

✓ 1 green tea bag or 1 teaspoon loose leaf green tea

✓ 1 cup hot water

- ✓ 1 tablespoon honey

- ✓ Juice of half a lemon

Instructions:

1. Steep the green tea in hot water for 3-5 minutes.

2. Remove the tea bag or strain the loose leaves.

3. Stir in honey and lemon juice.

4. Enjoy this refreshing, anti-inflammatory tea.

3. Chamomile and Peppermint Tea

Chamomile and peppermint together create a soothing, anti-inflammatory blend that's perfect for relaxing and reducing inflammation.

Ingredients:

- ✓ 1 chamomile tea bag or 1 tablespoon dried chamomile flowers

- ✓ 1 peppermint tea bag or 1 tablespoon dried peppermint leaves

- ✓ 2 cups hot water

Instructions:

1. Combine chamomile and peppermint in a teapot.

2. Pour hot water over the herbs and steep for 5-10 minutes.

3. Strain into cups.

4. Enjoy this calming and anti-inflammatory tea.

Anti-Inflammatory Tonics

1. Apple Cider Vinegar and Honey Tonic

Apple cider vinegar is known for its numerous health benefits, including its anti-inflammatory properties. This tonic is a great way to start your day.

Ingredients:

- ✓ 1 tablespoon apple cider vinegar

- ✓ 1 tablespoon honey

- ✓ 1 cup warm water

- ✓ A pinch of cinnamon (optional)

Instructions:

1. Mix apple cider vinegar and honey in a cup of warm water.

2. Stir well to combine.

3. Add a pinch of cinnamon for extra anti-inflammatory benefits.

4. Drink this tonic in the morning on an empty stomach.

2. Ginger Lemon Tonic

Ginger and lemon are both powerful anti-inflammatory agents. This tonic is not only refreshing but also great for digestion.

Ingredients:

- ✓ 1 tablespoon grated fresh ginger
- ✓ Juice of 1 lemon
- ✓ 1 tablespoon honey
- ✓ 2 cups hot water

Instructions:

1. Add grated ginger to a teapot with hot water.

2. Let steep for 10 minutes.

3. Strain into a cup and add lemon juice and honey.

4. Stir well and enjoy this invigorating tonic.

3. Golden Milk

Golden milk is a traditional Ayurvedic drink made with turmeric and milk (or a milk alternative). It's warming, soothing, and loaded with anti-inflammatory properties.

Ingredients:

- ✓ 1 cup almond milk or any milk alternative
- ✓ 1 teaspoon turmeric powder
- ✓ 1/2 teaspoon cinnamon
- ✓ 1/2 teaspoon ginger powder
- ✓ 1 tablespoon honey or maple syrup
- ✓ A pinch of black pepper

Instructions:

1. In a small pot, heat the almond milk over medium heat.

2. Add turmeric, cinnamon, ginger, honey, and black pepper.

3. Whisk to combine and heat until warm (do not boil).

4. Pour into a cup and enjoy this comforting, anti-inflammatory beverage.

Incorporating anti-inflammatory teas and tonics into your daily routine can be a delicious and effective way to manage gout and support overall health. From the golden richness of turmeric and ginger tea to the refreshing simplicity of green tea with lemon, these beverages are designed to provide relief and promote wellness. Experiment with these recipes and discover the soothing benefits of anti-inflammatory ingredients. Enjoy these drinks as part of your journey to better health and well-being.

10.3 Smoothies for Gout Relief

Smoothies are a convenient and delicious way to incorporate nutrient-dense foods into your diet. For those managing gout, certain ingredients can help reduce inflammation, promote hydration, and support overall health. In this section, we'll explore a variety of smoothie recipes specifically designed to provide relief from gout symptoms and enhance well-being.

Key Ingredients for Gout-Relieving Smoothies

When creating smoothies for gout relief, it's important to focus on ingredients that have anti-inflammatory properties, are low in purines, and support kidney function. Here are some key ingredients to include:

- ✓ **Berries:** Strawberries, blueberries, and cherries are rich in antioxidants and have anti-inflammatory properties.

- ✓ **Leafy Greens:** Spinach and kale are nutrient-dense and help reduce inflammation.

- ✓ **Citrus Fruits:** Oranges, lemons, and limes are high in vitamin C, which can help lower uric acid levels.

- ✓ **Low-Fat Dairy or Alternatives:** Yogurt and milk (or non-dairy alternatives like almond milk) provide essential nutrients without adding excess purines.

- ✓ **Ginger and Turmeric:** Both have strong anti-inflammatory properties.

- ✓ **Hydrating Ingredients:** Coconut water and cucumbers help maintain hydration, which is crucial for managing gout.

Gout-Relieving Smoothie Recipes

1. Berry Anti-Inflammatory Smoothie

This smoothie combines the anti-inflammatory power of berries with the hydrating benefits of coconut water.

Ingredients:

- ✓ 1 cup mixed berries (strawberries, blueberries, raspberries)
- ✓ 1/2 cup plain Greek yogurt or a dairy-free alternative
- ✓ 1/2 cup coconut water
- ✓ 1 tablespoon chia seeds
- ✓ 1 teaspoon honey or maple syrup (optional)
- ✓ Ice cubes (optional)

Instructions:

1. Combine all ingredients in a blender.
2. Blend until smooth.
3. Add ice cubes if desired for a colder smoothie.
4. Enjoy this refreshing and anti-inflammatory smoothie.

2. Green Detox Smoothie

This smoothie is packed with leafy greens and citrus fruits, making it a great choice for detoxifying and reducing inflammation.

Ingredients:

- ✓ 1 cup spinach or kale
- ✓ 1 green apple, chopped
- ✓ 1/2 cucumber, chopped
- ✓ Juice of 1 lemon
- ✓ 1/2 cup coconut water or plain water
- ✓ 1 tablespoon fresh ginger, grated
- ✓ 1 tablespoon honey or agave syrup (optional)
- ✓ Ice cubes (optional)

Instructions:

1. Combine all ingredients in a blender.
2. Blend until smooth.
3. Add ice cubes if desired for a colder smoothie.

4. Enjoy this nutrient-packed detox smoothie.

3. Citrus and Ginger Smoothie

This zesty smoothie is rich in vitamin C and ginger, providing a refreshing and anti-inflammatory boost.

Ingredients:

- ✓ 1 orange, peeled and segmented
- ✓ 1/2 cup pineapple chunks
- ✓ 1/2 banana
- ✓ 1/2 cup almond milk or any milk alternative
- ✓ 1 tablespoon fresh ginger, grated
- ✓ 1 tablespoon flaxseeds
- ✓ Ice cubes (optional)

Instructions:

1. Combine all ingredients in a blender.
2. Blend until smooth.
3. Add ice cubes if desired for a colder smoothie.
4. Enjoy this vibrant and tangy smoothie.

4. Cherry Almond Smoothie

Cherries are known for their gout-relieving properties, and this smoothie combines them with almonds for a delicious and nutritious drink.

Ingredients:

- ✓ 1 cup frozen cherries
- ✓ 1/2 cup almond milk
- ✓ 1/2 banana
- ✓ 1 tablespoon almond butter
- ✓ 1 tablespoon chia seeds
- ✓ 1 teaspoon vanilla extract
- ✓ Ice cubes (optional)

Instructions:

1. Combine all ingredients in a blender.
2. Blend until smooth.
3. Add ice cubes if desired for a colder smoothie.
4. Enjoy this sweet and satisfying smoothie.

5. Turmeric and Mango Smoothie

This tropical smoothie features turmeric for its anti-inflammatory benefits and mango for a sweet, refreshing flavor.

Ingredients:

- ✓ 1 cup frozen mango chunks
- ✓ 1/2 banana
- ✓ 1 cup almond milk or any milk alternative
- ✓ 1 teaspoon turmeric powder
- ✓ 1/2 teaspoon cinnamon
- ✓ 1 tablespoon honey or maple syrup (optional)
- ✓ Ice cubes (optional)

Instructions:

1. Combine all ingredients in a blender.
2. Blend until smooth.
3. Add ice cubes if desired for a colder smoothie.
4. Enjoy this tropical and anti-inflammatory smoothie.

Tips for Making the Perfect Gout-Relieving Smoothie

- ✓ **Balance Flavors:** Use a mix of sweet, tart, and creamy ingredients to create a balanced and enjoyable smoothie.

- ✓ **Adjust Consistency:** Add more liquid (water, coconut water, or milk) to thin out the smoothie or more frozen fruit/ice to thicken it.

- ✓ **Boost Nutrition:** Add superfoods like chia seeds, flaxseeds, or a handful of spinach to increase the nutritional value.

- ✓ **Stay Hydrated:** Incorporate hydrating ingredients like cucumber, coconut water, or water-rich fruits to support kidney function and overall hydration.

- ✓ **Listen to Your Body:** Everyone's body reacts differently to foods, so pay attention to how your body responds to certain ingredients and adjust accordingly.

Smoothies can be a delicious and effective way to manage gout and support overall health. By incorporating anti-inflammatory and hydrating ingredients, these smoothie recipes offer a convenient way to boost your nutrition and alleviate gout symptoms. Enjoy experimenting with these recipes and discover the benefits of adding gout-relieving smoothies to your daily routine.

CHAPTER ELEVEN
MEAL PLANS AND TIPS

11.1 7-Day Meal Plan for Gout Management

Managing gout effectively often requires a well-structured diet plan that helps control uric acid levels, reduces inflammation, and supports overall health. This 7-day meal plan is designed to provide you with a variety of delicious, gout-friendly meals that are easy to prepare and enjoy. Each day includes breakfast, lunch, dinner, and snacks to ensure balanced nutrition and satisfaction.

Day 1

Breakfast: Berry Smoothie Bowl

- ✓ 1 cup mixed berries (strawberries, blueberries, raspberries)

GOUT DIET COOKBOOK

- ✓ 1/2 cup plain Greek yogurt or a dairy-free alternative

- ✓ 1 tablespoon chia seeds

- ✓ 1 tablespoon honey (optional)

- ✓ Toppings: Sliced banana, almonds, and a drizzle of honey

Lunch: Quinoa and Vegetable Salad

- ✓ 1 cup cooked quinoa

- ✓ 1/2 cup cherry tomatoes, halved

- ✓ 1/2 cucumber, diced

- ✓ 1/4 cup feta cheese (optional)

- ✓ 2 tablespoons olive oil and lemon juice dressing

- ✓ Fresh herbs like parsley or mint

Dinner: Grilled Salmon with Steamed Vegetables

- ✓ 4 oz grilled salmon

- ✓ 1 cup steamed broccoli and carrots

- ✓ 1/2 cup brown rice

- ✓ Lemon wedges for garnish

Snack: Apple Slices with Almond Butter

- ✓ 1 apple, sliced

- ✓ 2 tablespoons almond butter

Day 2

Breakfast: Spinach and Mushroom Omelette

- ✓ 2 eggs or egg whites

- ✓ 1/2 cup spinach

- ✓ 1/4 cup sliced mushrooms

- ✓ 1 tablespoon olive oil

- ✓ Salt and pepper to taste

Lunch: Mediterranean Chickpea Salad

- ✓ 1 cup canned chickpeas, drained and rinsed

- ✓ 1/2 cup diced cucumbers

- ✓ 1/2 cup diced bell peppers

- ✓ 1/4 cup olives

- ✓ 2 tablespoons olive oil and red wine vinegar dressing

- ✓ Fresh basil

Dinner: Turkey and Vegetable Stir-Fry

- ✓ 4 oz ground turkey

- ✓ 1 cup mixed vegetables (bell peppers, snap peas, carrots)

- ✓ 1/2 cup brown rice

- ✓ 2 tablespoons low-sodium soy sauce

Snack: Greek Yogurt with Honey and Nuts

- ✓ 1/2 cup plain Greek yogurt

- ✓ 1 tablespoon honey

- ✓ 1 tablespoon chopped walnuts or almonds

Day 3

Breakfast: Oatmeal with Berries and Chia Seeds

- ✓ 1/2 cup rolled oats

- ✓ 1 cup almond milk

- ✓ 1/2 cup mixed berries

- ✓ 1 tablespoon chia seeds

- ✓ 1 tablespoon honey (optional)

Lunch: Lentil and Vegetable Soup

- ✓ 1 cup cooked lentils

- ✓ 1 cup mixed vegetables (carrots, celery, tomatoes)

- ✓ 2 cups vegetable broth

- ✓ 1/4 cup chopped parsley

Dinner: Baked Chicken with Sweet Potato and Green Beans

- ✓ 4 oz baked chicken breast

- ✓ 1 sweet potato, baked

- ✓ 1 cup steamed green beans

- ✓ Olive oil and herbs for seasoning

Snack: Carrot and Cucumber Sticks with Hummus

- ✓ 1/2 cup carrot sticks

- ✓ 1/2 cup cucumber sticks

- ✓ 1/4 cup hummus

Day 4

Breakfast: Avocado Toast with Cherry Tomatoes

- ✓ 1 slice whole-grain bread

- ✓ 1/2 avocado, mashed

- ✓ 1/4 cup cherry tomatoes, halved

- ✓ Salt, pepper, and a drizzle of olive oil

Lunch: Grilled Vegetable Wrap

- ✓ 1 whole-grain wrap

- ✓ 1/2 cup grilled zucchini and bell peppers

- ✓ 1/4 cup hummus

- ✓ Handful of spinach leaves

Dinner: Shrimp and Vegetable Skewers

- ✓ 4 oz shrimp, peeled and deveined

- ✓ 1 cup mixed vegetables (bell peppers, onions, cherry tomatoes)

- ✓ 1/2 cup quinoa

- ✓ Lemon wedges and fresh herbs for garnish

Snack: Mixed Nuts and Seeds

- ✓ 1/4 cup mixed nuts and seeds (almonds, walnuts, sunflower seeds)

Day 5

Breakfast: Smoothie with Spinach, Banana, and Almond Milk

- ✓ 1 cup almond milk
- ✓ 1 banana
- ✓ 1 cup spinach
- ✓ 1 tablespoon chia seeds
- ✓ 1 teaspoon honey (optional)

Lunch: Greek Salad with Chicken

- ✓ 4 oz grilled chicken breast
- ✓ 1 cup mixed greens

- ✓ 1/2 cup cherry tomatoes

- ✓ 1/4 cup olives

- ✓ 1/4 cup feta cheese (optional)

- ✓ 2 tablespoons olive oil and lemon juice dressing

Dinner: Stuffed Bell Peppers

- ✓ 2 bell peppers, halved and seeded

- ✓ 1 cup cooked quinoa

- ✓ 1/2 cup black beans

- ✓ 1/2 cup diced tomatoes

- ✓ 1/4 cup shredded cheese (optional)

Snack: Fresh Fruit Salad

- ✓ 1 cup mixed fresh fruits (pineapple, mango, berries)

Day 6

Breakfast: Chia Pudding with Berries

- ✓ 3 tablespoons chia seeds

- ✓ 1 cup almond milk

- ✓ 1/2 cup mixed berries

GOUT DIET COOKBOOK

- ✓ 1 teaspoon honey (optional)

Lunch: Tuna and White Bean Salad

- ✓ 1 can tuna, drained

- ✓ 1 cup canned white beans, drained and rinsed

- ✓ 1/2 cup diced cucumbers

- ✓ 1/4 cup red onion, diced

- ✓ 2 tablespoons olive oil and lemon juice dressing

Dinner: Baked Cod with Asparagus

- ✓ 4 oz baked cod

- ✓ 1 cup roasted asparagus

- ✓ 1/2 cup wild rice

- ✓ Lemon wedges for garnish

Snack: Celery Sticks with Peanut Butter

- ✓ 1/2 cup celery sticks

- ✓ 2 tablespoons peanut butter

Day 7

Breakfast: Whole-Grain Pancakes with Fresh Berries

GOUT DIET COOKBOOK

- ✓ 1/2 cup whole-grain pancake mix

- ✓ 1/2 cup almond milk

- ✓ 1/2 cup fresh berries

- ✓ 1 tablespoon maple syrup

Lunch: Quinoa and Black Bean Bowl

- ✓ 1 cup cooked quinoa

- ✓ 1/2 cup black beans

- ✓ 1/2 cup diced bell peppers

- ✓ 1/4 cup corn

- ✓ 2 tablespoons salsa

Dinner: Roasted Chicken with Root Vegetables

- ✓ 4 oz roasted chicken breast

- ✓ 1 cup mixed root vegetables (carrots, parsnips, sweet potatoes)

- ✓ 1/2 cup brown rice

- ✓ Olive oil and herbs for seasoning

Snack: Cottage Cheese with Pineapple

- ✓ 1/2 cup cottage cheese

✓ 1/2 cup pineapple chunks

Tips for Success

✓ **Plan Ahead:** Take some time at the beginning of the week to plan your meals, make a grocery list, and prep ingredients. This will save you time and reduce stress during the week.

✓ **Batch Cook:** Prepare larger portions of meals like soups, stews, and quinoa, and store them in the refrigerator or freezer for quick and easy meals later in the week.

✓ **Stay Hydrated:** Drink plenty of water throughout the day to help flush uric acid from your system. Aim for at least 8 cups of water daily.

✓ **Listen to Your Body:** Pay attention to how your body responds to different foods. Everyone's experience with gout is unique, so adjust your diet as needed based on what works best for you.

✓ **Incorporate Variety:** Enjoy a wide range of fruits, vegetables, lean proteins, and whole grains to ensure you're getting a balanced diet full of essential nutrients.

GOUT DIET COOKBOOK

- ✓ **Moderation is Key:** While it's important to avoid high-purine foods, remember that moderation is key. Enjoying a diverse diet will help you avoid feeling deprived and make it easier to stick to your meal plan.

- ✓ **Stay Active:** Regular physical activity can help manage gout symptoms and improve overall health. Aim for at least 30 minutes of moderate exercise most days of the week.

- ✓ **Seek Support:** Consider working with a nutritionist or joining a support group for people with gout. Sharing experiences and tips can provide motivation and new ideas for managing your condition.

Following a well-balanced meal plan tailored to managing gout can make a significant difference in your quality of life. By incorporating a variety of nutrient-rich, low-purine foods and staying hydrated, you can help reduce gout symptoms and improve overall health. This 7-day meal plan offers a delicious and practical approach to eating well while managing gout. Enjoy experimenting with these recipes and make them your own as you discover what works best for you.

11.2 Tips for Eating Out with Gout

Eating out while managing gout can be challenging, but it doesn't have to be a daunting experience. With a bit of planning and mindful choices, you can enjoy dining out without triggering a gout flare-up. Here are some practical tips to help you navigate restaurant menus and make gout-friendly choices.

Plan Ahead

Research the Menu: Before heading out, check the restaurant's menu online. Look for options that align with your dietary needs and identify potential triggers to avoid. Many restaurants now provide detailed nutritional information, which can be helpful in making informed choices.

Call Ahead: Don't hesitate to call the restaurant in advance to ask about specific ingredients or preparation methods. This can also give you an opportunity to request modifications to menu items to make them more gout-friendly.

Make Smart Choices

GOUT DIET COOKBOOK

Choose Lean Proteins: Opt for lean protein sources like chicken, turkey, or fish. Avoid red meats and organ meats, which are high in purines and can trigger gout attacks. Grilled, baked, or steamed preparations are generally healthier choices than fried or sautéed options.

Load Up on Vegetables: Vegetables are your best friends when managing gout. Look for dishes that feature plenty of fresh or cooked vegetables. Salads, steamed veggies, and vegetable-based soups are excellent choices. Avoid vegetables that are fried or cooked in heavy sauces.

Whole Grains: Choose whole grains like brown rice, quinoa, or whole-wheat pasta over refined grains. These options provide more fiber and nutrients, which are beneficial for overall health.

Watch the Sauces and Dressings: Many sauces and dressings can be high in purines, sodium, or unhealthy fats. Ask for these on the side, so you can control the amount you use. Opt for olive oil and vinegar for salads, or a simple lemon squeeze for added flavor.

Mindful Dining

Portion Control: Restaurant portions can be large, so consider sharing a meal with a friend or asking for a half portion. You can also box up half of your meal at the start to avoid overeating.

Stay Hydrated: Drink plenty of water throughout your meal. Staying hydrated helps flush uric acid from your system and can prevent gout flare-ups. Avoid sugary drinks and limit alcohol consumption, as both can increase uric acid levels.

Pace Yourself: Take your time eating and savor each bite. Eating slowly can help you recognize when you're full and prevent overeating.

Specific Cuisine Tips

Italian: Choose tomato-based sauces over cream-based ones. Opt for grilled fish or chicken dishes, and avoid heavy pasta dishes with rich, creamy sauces. A vegetable-based minestrone soup is a great starter.

Chinese: Go for steamed dishes like steamed vegetables, tofu, or fish. Avoid fried items and dishes with heavy sauces. Brown rice is a better choice than white rice. Look for stir-fried dishes that are not overly greasy.

Mexican: Choose dishes with lean proteins and plenty of vegetables. Skip the fried tortilla chips and opt for salsa or guacamole as a dip. A chicken or vegetable fajita with whole-wheat tortillas is a good option.

Indian: Select tandoori (grilled) meats and vegetable-based curries. Avoid dishes with heavy cream sauces like korma or masala. Dal (lentil) dishes and chana masala (chickpeas) are excellent choices.

Japanese: Sushi can be a healthy option, but avoid high-purine fish like mackerel or herring. Opt for vegetable rolls, cucumber rolls, or California rolls. Miso soup and seaweed salad are also good choices.

Communicate Your Needs

Speak Up: Don't be afraid to ask your server about how dishes are prepared or to request modifications. Most restaurants are willing to accommodate dietary restrictions if you explain your needs politely.

Custom Orders: Feel free to customize your order to better fit your dietary needs. For example, you can ask for grilled chicken instead of fried, or request extra vegetables in place of starchy sides.

Enjoy the Experience

Focus on the Company: Remember that dining out is not just about the food but also about the experience and the company. Enjoy the social aspect of your meal and focus on the pleasure of being with friends or family.

Treat Yourself: While it's important to stick to a gout-friendly diet, it's also okay to treat yourself occasionally. Just be mindful of portion sizes and balance indulgences with healthy choices.

Eating out with gout doesn't have to be restrictive or stressful. By planning ahead, making smart choices, and communicating your needs, you can enjoy dining out while managing your condition effectively. Remember, the goal is to maintain a balanced diet that supports your health and well-being. Enjoy your meals and the dining experience, knowing that you can make choices that help keep your gout under control.

11.3 Staying on Track: Long-Term Strategies

Managing gout requires a long-term commitment to making healthy lifestyle choices. By incorporating these strategies into your daily routine, you can effectively control uric acid levels, reduce inflammation, and prevent gout flare-ups over the long term.

Commit to a Balanced Diet

Consistency is Key: Stick to a balanced diet that focuses on whole grains, lean proteins, plenty of fruits and vegetables, and healthy fats. Avoid or limit foods high in purines, saturated fats, and refined sugars.

Portion Control: Pay attention to portion sizes to prevent overeating, which can contribute to weight gain and increased uric acid levels. Use smaller plates and bowls to help control portion sizes.

Stay Hydrated: Drink plenty of water throughout the day to help flush uric acid from your system. Aim for at least 8-10 cups of water daily. Avoid sugary drinks and limit alcohol consumption, as both can increase uric acid levels.

GOUT DIET COOKBOOK

Maintain a Healthy Weight

Achieve and Maintain a Healthy Weight: Maintaining a healthy weight can help reduce uric acid levels and lower your risk of gout attacks. Aim for gradual, sustainable weight loss if you are overweight or obese.

Regular Exercise: Engage in regular physical activity to support overall health and manage gout symptoms. Aim for at least 150 minutes of moderate-intensity aerobic activity, such as brisk walking or cycling, each week.

Include Strength Training: Incorporate strength training exercises into your routine to build muscle mass and improve joint stability. This can help support your joints and reduce the risk of gout flare-ups.

Monitor Your Uric Acid Levels

Regular Monitoring: Work with your healthcare provider to monitor your uric acid levels regularly. This can help track your progress and make adjustments to your treatment plan as needed.

Medication Adherence: If prescribed medication to manage gout, take it as directed by your healthcare provider. This can help prevent gout attacks and reduce the risk of complications associated with high uric acid levels.

Stress Management

Practice Stress-Relief Techniques: Chronic stress can trigger gout attacks in some individuals. Incorporate stress-relief techniques such as mindfulness meditation, deep breathing exercises, yoga, or hobbies that you enjoy.

Lifestyle Adjustments

Avoid Triggers: Identify and avoid triggers that may contribute to gout flare-ups, such as certain foods (high-purine foods, sugary beverages), alcohol, and dehydration.

Educate Yourself: Stay informed about gout management strategies and new research developments. Knowledge empowers you to make informed decisions about your health.

Build a Support Network

Seek Support: Connect with others who are managing gout or chronic conditions. Support groups or online communities can provide encouragement, practical tips, and emotional support.

Involve Your Family: Educate your family members about gout and how they can support you in managing your condition. Encourage healthy eating habits for the whole family.

Long-Term Mindset

Set Realistic Goals: Set achievable goals for yourself and celebrate your successes along the way. Long-term management of gout requires dedication and persistence.

Be Patient: Managing gout is a journey that may involve ups and downs. Be patient with yourself and stay committed to making positive lifestyle changes.

By adopting these long-term strategies, you can effectively manage gout and improve your quality of life. Consistently following a balanced diet, maintaining a healthy weight, staying active, monitoring uric acid levels, managing stress, and building a support network are key components of long-term gout management. With dedication and a proactive approach, you can minimize gout flare-ups and enjoy a healthier, more active lifestyle.

CONCLUSION

In conclusion, managing gout through dietary choices can significantly impact your quality of life by reducing flare-ups and promoting overall health. This Gout Diet Cookbook has been crafted to provide you with delicious and nutritious recipes that support your journey towards managing gout effectively.

Through the pages of this cookbook, you've explored a variety of meal options designed to be low in purines, rich in essential nutrients, and satisfying to the palate. From flavorful breakfast smoothies to hearty dinners and indulgent yet safe desserts, each recipe has been thoughtfully selected to help you enjoy meals without compromising on taste or health.

Beyond recipes, we've discussed the importance of understanding gout, the role of diet in managing symptoms, and practical tips for grocery shopping, meal planning, and eating out. By embracing a balanced diet that includes plenty of fruits, vegetables, lean proteins, and whole grains while limiting high-purine foods, you can proactively support your gout management goals.

Remember, managing gout is a journey that requires commitment, patience, and a proactive approach to health. By incorporating the principles and recipes from this cookbook into your daily routine, you are taking positive steps towards not only managing gout but also enjoying a vibrant and fulfilling life.

Whether you are just starting on your journey or seeking new ways to enhance your current gout management plan, let this cookbook be your guide to delicious meals that nourish your body and support your well-being. Here's to good health and flavorful eating!

THANKS FOR YOUR ATTENTION!!!